A TIME TO HEAL

I should have died of malignant melanoma, one of the fastest-spreading cancers, around June 1981. Today I am healthy in the full sense of the word; not just not-ill but enjoying great well-being and energy. When my secondary cancer was diagnosed in late 1980, I was also suffering from diabetes, incipient osteo-arthritis, frequent knockout migraines and chronic dental abscesses. All those ailments have vanished; it is as if I had been granted a second youth. A large part of my right leg, mutilated by cancer surgery, has grown back. Doctor friends assure me that such regeneration is impossible and I believe them – except that I happen to walk on that impossibility every day of my life.

Alongside my physical recovery, I have also undergone an inner transformation that has stripped away many of my fears, burdens and obsolete values, leaving me with a sense of increased freedom and wholeness. I worry much less and laugh much more than I did in the past. But once you have travelled to the edge of death and then returned to a life more abundant, your ability to worry simply melts away.

About the Author

Beata Bishop is a writer and psychotherapist, working along Jungian and Transpersonal lines. After a cosmopolitan upbringing she has spent most of her life in London, except for residing briefly in Canada and France and travelling extensively all over Europe. She has worked as a journalist and spent eleven years writing radio scripts for the BBC.

When her secondary cancer struck and orthodox medicine had very little to offer, she turned to the alternative field and chose the Gerson therapy to which she now attributes her survival and her present health and vitality.

A TIME TO HEAL

BEATA BISHOP

Triumph over cancer
The therapy of the future

NEW ENGLISH LIBRARY
Hodder and Stoughton

Copyright © Beata Bishop 1985

First published in Great Britain in
1985 by Severn House Publishers Ltd

First New English Library paperback
edition 1989

British Library C.I.P.

Bishop, Beata
    A time to heal: triumph over
cancer. the therapy of the future.
1. Man. Cancer. Therapy
I. Title
616.99'406

ISBN 0-450-50085-3

Printed and bound in Great Britain
for Hodder and Stoughton
paperbacks, a division of Hodder and
Stoughton Ltd, Mill Road,
Dunton Green, Sevenoaks, Kent
TN13 2YA (Editorial Office: 47 Bedford
Square, London WC1B 3DP) by R. Clay
Ltd, Bungay, Suffolk.

This book is dedicated with love and gratitude to all those who helped me to recover, and to the memory of Dr Max Gerson.

Publisher's note

This book is in no way a guide to the Gerson therapy.
It is a story of one woman's experience, *not* an outline
of the workings of the therapy. The publishers stress
that anyone interested in the therapy should contact
The Gerson Institute, P O box 430, Bonita, California
92002 USA: Telephone: (619) 267 1150, which will give
any information that might be required. The author
regrets she is unable to deal with enquiries.

Contents

Foreword

Dr S. J. L. Mount, MB, BS, MRCP, FFHom.

I HAVE KNOWN Beata Bishop for thirteen years and, having followed her progress through the past few incredible years, can vouch in every way for what is recorded in these pages regarding her cure. Beata is now completely free of cancer, and this as a result of the Gerson therapy she underwent. Not only is she free of cancer, she is free of malignant melanoma, one of the fastest spreading cancers. Her story is exciting and challenging from a personal point of view but is also medically fascinating and stimulating in every way. Cancer can be cured. It is a question of the right approach.

In 1977, with my wife I visited the Gerson clinic in Tijuana, where Beata Bishop was treated in 1981, and I was shown round by the daughter of Dr Gerson, Charlotte Gerson Straus, who is now the greatest living expert in the cancer treatments pioneered by her late father. The clinic was full of cancer patients, many of whom spoke of remarkable progress on the therapy. The visit was one of the highlights of my career and the clinic is a remarkable tribute to the energy, enthusiasm and brilliance of Charlotte Gerson Straus in the drive to cure cancer.

In his book, *A Cancer Therapy – Results of Fifty Cases*, Dr Gerson explains the rationale behind his therapy, which is basically to alter the body's sodium-potassium balance by flooding the body with potassium ions, richly contained in juices, raw vegetables and fruits. The body is detoxified and elimination stimulated by enemas, and the basic metabolism is adjusted with small amounts of thyroid, liver and certain vitamins. That this treatment is successful in many cases is borne out by the fifty cases outlined in Gerson's own book, and by recent cases documented by Charlotte Gerson Straus in her periodic reports from the clinic. In that sense Beata Bishop is one of a long line of cured patients. The Gerson therapy must stand as one of the most successful of all natural therapies in the treatment of cancer; certainly it is the most consistent regarding methodology, regime and results.

In fact, the regime is tough to follow, and not for the faint-hearted. Courage, persistence and, above all, faith are required at all stages. The preparation of the many juices, the gathering of organic vegetables and fruit, the making of special potassium solutions and, above all, the frequent application of enemas, consume a great deal of time and energy. The therapy is hard work. Frequently the body goes through certain healing crises, particularly if drugs have been taken or there has been a history of poor nutrition, or, again, if metastases or tissue necrosis have occurred. These stages of healing can be painful.

Anybody who knows Beata well recognises in her the qualities of courage, persistence and faith necessary to carry the treatments through. Her book testifies to this and to her tremendous determination to survive, to live and to be cured. I feel indeed privileged to contribute a foreword to this book and only hope that others may be inspired to follow this way of cure and learn from Beata Bishop's rich experience.

Dr S. J. L. Mount

Introduction to This Edition

FOUR YEARS HAVE passed since this book was first published. In the jaunty phrase of my Mexican surgeon friend, I am still 'beating the statistics', being alive and remarkably well, with ample energy and *joie de vivre*. Recently an osteopath, whom I consulted after an over-ambitious yoga session, read out to me a long checklist of complaints and symptoms which, he explained, middle-aged people tend to have. I had none. Since he seemed astonished, I suggested that lifestyle might be more relevant than chronological age, and when I described mine, he agreed.

Not that I lead an ascetic existence. Since coming off the therapy in early 1983, I have been careful to avoid junk food and other harmful substances, and I live largely on an organically produced lacto-vegetarian diet, occasionally adding some fish or chicken. Much of the time I follow the Gerson diet fairly closely, because I thrive on it; every now and then I break the rules with glee, and that suits me too.

As a wisecracking friend once said, anyone who recovers from cancer *and* survives the rigours of the intensive Gerson therapy should live for ever. Well, not quite. But we should have a good long innings.

Cancer still plays a large, if indirect, role in my life and I suspect it always will. As soon as I ceased to be a patient, I became a helper through a spontaneous role reversal that overtakes many former sufferers, as if the past experience of cancer obliged us to stay in the field and give support to others. There is nothing noble or

11

premeditated about this. It arises naturally, like all loyalties born from shared suffering. How much I can do for others varies a great deal, but most of the unknown cancer patients who ring me out of the blue to ask questions, compare notes or ask for counselling seem to derive comfort from my survival against heavy odds, just as I once found hope in other patients' recovery, since nothing is more encouraging than to hear that someone has managed to climb the dreadful mountain on which you are stranded halfway, in a thick fog.

Going beyond the purely personal, I can see some positive changes that have occurred in the cancer field over the past few years, especially in the non-medical sector. It is lay people who set up cancer support groups and self-help centres – and then often wait in vain for local GPs to refer patients to them. It is lay people who train and work as counsellors or befrienders to cancer sufferers, and who compile and spread information on nutrition and other alternative techniques, having first tried and tested them. Above all, it is among lay people that cancer is discussed more openly than ever before, which is the essential first step towards de-mystifying the disease and taking responsibility for one's own health and well-being.

In the medical field, the positive changes are less obvious. True, some doctors have become more receptive to unconventional approaches. Many acknowledge the value of nurse-counsellors (but have no funds to employ them), and others are in favour of healers (provided they know their place). The 1981 report by Sir Richard Doll and Richard Peto, which established that dietary factors were the main *single* cause of cancer, outstripping even tobacco, has brought nutrition in from the cold, but only as a means of prevention. The official line now runs that the right diet can help to *prevent* cancer, but once the malignant disease has struck, diet cannot make any difference.

I have read this demonstrably untrue opinion many times in the Press and heard it on radio and TV. Worst of all, I have even had it expressed to me by several doctors whom I wanted to interest in the life-saving potential of the Gerson therapy. Surely, I thought, they would want to explore a method that could help their own patients; surely my own highly unusual recovery would at least whet their curiosity.

But I was wrong. With two exceptions all the doctors whom I approached chose to make categorical statements rather than ask questions, so that our conversations ended before they could have properly begun.

One doctor, for instance, informed me that mine had been a spontaneous recovery which was not at all unusual – really, there was no point in discussing it any further. (Oddly enough, spontaneous recovery is only ever ascribed to patients who regain their health by unorthodox means.)

Another one said that as cancer is incurable, I was only in remission and would relapse sooner or later. I did not consider that statement particularly helpful, although it did not worry me. More importantly, at the time of our meeting, I had survived for seven years since starting on the Gerson therapy, and according to the well-known medical rule, five years' survival equals a cure. (Strangely enough, this only seems to apply to conventionally treated patients.)

A third doctor expressed the view that I must have recovered despite that weird therapy.

A fourth dismissed the Gerson therapy as unscientific and added that after the excision of my original tumour, I should have also had a batch of healthy lymph glands removed, undergone massive radiation, and then hoped for the best. When I quietly suggested that hoping for the best was not very scientific, he got quite annoyed.

A fifth doctor, told of my case by a mutual acquaintance, said, 'She might just as well have gone to Lourdes'.

13

I did, however, have a courteous hearing from two eminent consultants who found my story interesting – and then dismissed it as anecdotal evidence, i.e. worthless.

All of this has made me sad; sometimes angry; sometimes both. But, although a handful of people have accused me of an anti-medicine bias, my negative feelings are not against doctors. Many of my early heroes were physicians and at one time I wanted to take up medicine myself. My anger is certainly not against the medical profession. But I dread and passionately oppose the bullying, patronising, superior attitude that refuses to listen, that dismisses out of hand anything new or unfamiliar and relies on hereditary professional authority to make its views prevail. In brief, I am against what Herbert Spencer called 'the principle of condemnation before investigation', which, he added, 'cannot fail to keep a man in everlasting ignorance'.

However, all is not gloom. Since 1983, a group of surgeons at the big District Hospital of Graz, in Austria, has been conducting a clinical trial of a watered-down version of the Gerson therapy on sixty patients suffering from a wide variety of cancers, many of them with secondaries in the liver. An interim report shows that even this emasculated Gerson programme, followed by patients in their own homes under medical supervision, brings above-average results. The Gerson patients of Graz live longer, feel better, need fewer drugs, show more optimism and suffer few, if any, side effects of the chemotherapy many of them also receive. The Austrian doctors monitoring the trial freely admit that they are conservative, sceptical and out of sympathy with 'so-called alternative methods' – none of which stops them from observing and assessing the results of the experiment, or from trying to understand why the Gerson therapy might work.

This is all anyone, in fairness, can ask of any doctor.

So far only the team in Graz has responded to the challenge. But that is an important first step.

Meanwhile in the United States independent medical authorities are reviewing the fully documented case histories of twenty cancer patients who have recovered solely on the Gerson therapy, despite a very poor outlook in each case. At the time of writing those independent experts, all high-ranking Establishment figures, are scrutinising the X-rays, CAT-scans, biopsy slides and pathology reports of the twenty 'best cases' submitted by the Gerson Institute. Their reports will be presented to the US Congressional Office of Technology Assessment, as part of an investigation into alternative cancer therapies. A great deal depends on the outcome of that presentation.

As one of the twenty 'best cases', I have a special interest in the matter.

Beata Bishop
London 1988

Introduction to the First Edition

I SHOULD HAVE died of malignant melanoma, one of the fastest-spreading cancers, around June 1981. Today I am healthy in the full sense of the word; not just not-ill but enjoying great well-being and energy. When my secondary cancer was diagnosed in late 1980, I was also suffering from diabetes, incipient osteo-arthritis, frequent knockout migraines and chronic dental abscesses. All those ailments have vanished; it is as if I had been granted a second youth. A large part of my right leg, mutilated by cancer surgery, has grown back. Doctor friends assure me that such regeneration is impossible and I believe them – except that I happen to walk on that impossibility every day of my life.

Alongside my physical recovery, I have also undergone an inner transformation that has stripped away many of my fears, burdens and obsolete values, leaving me with a sense of increased freedom and wholeness. I worry much less and laugh much more than I did in the past. But once you have travelled to the edge of death and then returned to a life more abundant, your ability to worry simply melts away.

My journey from life-threatening disease to health was not a free trip. It cost me eighteen months of close confinement on a tough, monotonous therapy that consumed most of my time and energy. It cost me my job and a great deal of money. It destroyed my lifestyle and forced me into an earthy, body-centred existence a world away from my former mode of being that had been airy, colourful and focussed on the things of the mind. The journey also demolished my long-held self-image and through a series of inner upheavals forced me to take a fresh look at myself and acknowledge my shadow. Last but not least, I had to endure many spells of vile sickness, pain, depression and weakness, the dark night of the soul and body when not being born seemed an irresistible lost opportunity.

Yet despite the high cost I would not have missed the experience. It has taught me lessons that might have otherwise taken several lifetimes to learn.

One of the toughest aspects of the process was its loneliness. I recovered on the Gerson therapy, which is an unorthodox nutritional programme, and backed it with some equally unorthodox physical and psychological techniques. Neither the National Health Service nor private health insurance companies recognise alternative therapies, so that if you choose one, you are on your own both financially and in terms of medical support. My own recovery was a strictly do-it-yourself job, except for the first two months which I spent at the world's only Gerson clinic in Mexico. Over the following sixteen months I battled on at home, helped by friends, supervised by a sympathetic physician and advised over the telephone or in writing by the late Dr Gerson's daughter, Charlotte, in California, or by his grand-daughter, Margaret, in London. Even with that support system the process was chillingly lonely, although having to take responsibility for your own survival or death is a splendid aid to growing up at any age.

What made the loneliness worse was that when my illness reached crisis point, alternative medicine was still a largely suspect minority cult, not a topic of wide public interest as it is today: alternative cancer treatments were practically unknown. If you stepped off the orthodox path, there was nowhere to go for support, advice or referral. Today, the Bristol Cancer Help Centre is nationally known and other centres, information

17

points and self-help groups are springing up every-where. But at the time all you could rely on was luck and the helpfulness of like-minded people who passed you along a rudimentary grapevine until you found the information you needed.

I wrote this account of my experience because I believe that what happened to me is relevant far beyond my individual fate. My own survival, much as I enjoy it, is of no consequence outside my small personal world. But it is important as a case history, because it proves that, against all expectations, a highly unconventional, though medically sound therapy has succeeded once more, as it has done so often over the years, largely in the United States, and can do so again and again, given a proper chance. At a time when one in four people die of cancer in the Western world – in 1936 the rate was one in fourteen – and when the survival figures of the most widespread cancers have not improved for thirty-five years, such a therapy cannot be ignored.

This book is a personal story, not a do-it-yourself cancer cure manual (but there is a book list at the end for further reading, and a brief summary on how to use food for disease prevention). Although my life was saved by the Gerson therapy, I do not claim that it is the only alternative cancer treatment that works, only that it has the longest and best track record. Besides, most other unorthodox therapies are based on the Gerson diet. It is true that the intensive therapy is demanding, hard and boring, with a correspondingly high drop-out rate; no one can see it through without strong motivation, patience and perseverance. If anyone ever produces an easier and faster version that works just as well, I shall be the first to cheer loudly.

It is also true that the therapy is no panacea and carries no guarantee of a cure. No therapy does. What matters is that it views health and disease from a fresh, revolutionary angle which is still waiting to be discovered and understood by orthodox medicine. (If Dr Gerson had not been some fifty years ahead of his time, he would not have had such a rough ride.) It is the originality and wide sweep of Gerson's thinking that explains why his therapy cures not only cancer but, with some modifications, also many other chronic degenerative diseases which are considered incurable at present, ranging from heart and kidney problems to multiple sclerosis and Alzheimer's Disease. Today, when these chronic diseases are fast outstripping our medical resources, we cannot afford to disregard the evidence of alternative therapy.

At present, it is hard to see when alternative therapies will come into their own. Western medicine is passing through a strange, mixed-up period of uncertainty and crises of both cash and confidence, with changes surfacing so fast that whatever one observes today may be out of date by next month. The lay alternative camp has long urged a move away from the current mechanistic, high technology, over-drugged, drastically interventionist and symptom-centred medicine towards a holistic, gentle and natural kind that concentrates on causes, not symptoms; a medicine in which the patient, acknowledged to consist of body, mind, feelings and spirit, is an equal partner in the healing process, not a passive pawn to whom things are done. Now some doctors have begun to say the same – in public, too. In September 1983, they set up the British Holistic Medical Association to further those aims. (A similar organisation has been functioning in the United States for ten years.) At present, these doctors are in a small minority. And, naturally, any change in direction will be fought by the majority. It cannot be otherwise. Doctors are the products of their training and of the brainwashing practised by the rich and powerful drug industry (which is also behind the charities conducting research into intractable chronic diseases – a line-up that effectively blocks any new departure that might clash with the interests of the drug lobby). For doctors to adopt a radically new approach, especially in cancer medicine, would equal the admission of having followed the wrong track all their lives. Can any ordinary human being be expected to do that without fierce resistance?

Meanwhile, outside the medical citadel, lay people and alternative therapists are asking new questions about the nature of cancer and of the human being who develops it. At a handful of centres doctors offer alternative treatments, but the field is desperately short of funds and facilities, and new methods can only be tested, researched, taught and practised in a small, resource-starved way. Official funds are not forthcoming because alternative practitioners have not produced sufficient scientific evidence to support their claims, and they cannot produce the evidence because of lack of funds. Thus the vicious circle spins on.

The alternative camp itself is far from unanimous in its approach to healing cancer. Some therapies, headed by the Gerson programme, focus on restoring the body through diet and detoxification and do little else. Others, like the Simonton visualisation technique, ignore diet and only stimulate the patient's will and imagination to promote physical and mental improvement. Yet other approaches lean strongly towards the psychological and spiritual aspects of healing, adding the physical more or less as an afterthought. Personally, I believe that the truly holistic approach which takes into account the body, mind, emotions and spirit is most likely to succeed; an approach which mobilises inner resources and heals psychological wounds while paying equal attention to the ravaged liver or bankrupt immune system that is also part of the pattern.

This approach is still being evolved out of trial and error, observation and intuition, caring and an open mind. There are plenty of traps, snags and tripwires along the way; most of the work is still waiting to be done.

This book is my contribution to that work.

Beata Bishop
London 1985

1

I DO NOT know when the brown spot first appeared on my right shin, roughly halfway between the knee and the ankle and slightly off centre. It may have been some time in the mid-seventies, but I did not notice its early beginnings. What I did notice at some unspecified moment was that it was there, and then, much later, that it was slowly growing in area, though not changing in any other way. I watched it carefully for changes in its colour, texture or thickness which, I knew from cancer prevention leaflets, might herald danger. But my brown spot was not changing, nor did it remotely resemble a mole or a sore. It was just a piece of cappuccino-coloured skin, normal and smooth, expanding slowly.

It did not worry me, my brown spot. I checked it daily in the bath, and only half a dozen times over a period of three years or more did I ask myself, lightly, whether it could possibly be melanoma (about which I knew only that it was a fast-spreading skin cancer which could be fatal). But the inner voice that had asked that question had been different from the normal one which I used to discuss things with myself. It had come from an unknown area of my consciousness and so I had dismissed it. In due course, the spot grew to the size of an irregularly shaped fingernail, but it was not unsightly. A friend who noticed it even thought that it looked sexy, in the manner of a far-flung beauty spot. I could not have thought of a nicer interpretation myself.

My general health caused me no worry, either. I was

23

fitter in middle age than I had been in my youth, with good energy and high resistance to infections. During a 'flu epidemic that had laid low most of my colleagues, I worked in dull solitude at the end of a depopulated office corridor, half-wishing I had caught the bug, too, rather than holding the fort alone. But then, unlike my colleagues – I was a BBC scriptwriter at the time – I followed a regime which some considered healthy and others thought cranky or worse; either way it worked for me. I lived on a lacto-vegetarian diet and avoided junk foods. I also avoided orthodox medicine whenever possible, and consulted an excellent medical herbalist rather than my local GP (who looked like an undertaker and prescribed either soluble aspirin or antibiotics). I also went to yoga classes, and although yoga is strictly non-competitive, it pleased me that I was more flexible than many women half my age. All in all, I was satisfied with my physical condition – when I thought about it, which was not often. To me my body was the vehicle I rode in. It seemed adequate, so I did not bother much about it.

What did worry me more and more was my inability to stop smoking. That was a problem and a burden on my conscience, for smoking did not fit in with my self-image or lifestyle. It seemed illogical to cultivate good health through diet and exercise and then damage it with nicotine. Also, what was that expensive, smelly dependence doing in my life when I was busy striving, or so I thought, to achieve inner freedom? Besides, how could I justify polluting everybody else's air space? But none of these arguments helped. My addiction to cigarettes was irrational, so I could not very well reason myself out of it. At least I did not cough, huff and puff – my yoga breathing exercises saw to that – and one day, I promised myself, I would give up anyway.

That was the general picture in November 1979, when I went for a routine check-up to Dr Ailsa Hay, the gynaecologist who had been looking after me for some years. I was glad to see her again. She was friendly, warm and caring, a fellow woman who happened to be a doctor, not the other way round. We had our usual preliminary chat and then continued with the conversation while she examined me on the narrow couch; always an apprehensive moment because, of course, she might find a lump in my breast or some ominous irregularity elsewhere that had not been there before ('There's always a first time', our old family doctor used to say lugubriously,) and what then?

But instead of announcing some potential gynaecological doom, Dr Hay only asked me whether 'that thing' on my leg was giving me any trouble.

'What thing?' I craned my neck and found Dr Hay contemplating the brown spot on my leg. 'Oh; that . . .' I began but stopped, because in the strong beam of her spotlight the spot looked different. It looked disturbed, no longer smooth and sealed but with an angry purple spot pushing up in its middle, breaking through the skin. It was not like anything I had seen before but, absurdly, it reminded me of an image from a recent dream of mine in which two large paving stones were being pushed up by some mysterious dark force rising from the earth below. When had the spot begun the change? Why had I not noticed it before? Or had I unconsciously chosen not to notice it?

'Does it ever hurt or bleed?' Dr Hay asked.

'No, never. What on earth can it be?'

'I don't know. But if I had something like that on my leg, I'd go and see a skin specialist at once.'

'All right,' I said. 'If you would, I will, too.' I got dressed, puzzled by this unexpected twist. Dr Hay was already writing a note to Dr Colville, an eminent dermatologist whom she knew well – 'He trains all the young ones,' she added – and advised me to see him soon. As we parted, she seemed more concerned than I. Walking away from her premises, I kept gazing at my right leg with its no longer familiar spot. Could it be a leg ulcer, I wondered, not knowing what that looked like, either. But I felt sure it was nothing serious and I hurried on to the office to grapple with my Christmas programme script.

Dr Colville, the eminent dermatologist, saw me four days later. He was a tall, elegant man, well into his sixties, wearing a superbly tailored suit, a sumptuous silk tie and gleaming shoes. As I was shown in, he was leaning against an antique cabinet in the pose of a distinguished actor playing a distinguished medical man. In fact, what struck me most, beside the perfection of his clothes, was his dated theatrical manner. The way he smiled and moved forward with small, fast, fluttering movements, the way he gestured and made me sit down with a flourish of cuffs suggested that he might suddenly burst into a song and dance routine, providing the Harley Street version of the late Maurice Chevalier. I wondered what kind of a *persona* he projected in the general ward of an ordinary hospital.

He read Dr Hay's letter, said, 'She's a good girl,' blinked at me as if I had just materialised out of nowhere and asked me to show him my leg. He, too, shone a strong spotlight on it for a few seconds before saying, 'That'll have to come out.'

'Why?'

'Because in two or three years' time it might cause you a lot of trouble. Better get rid of it now and live happily ever after. What are you doing over Christmas?'

'Nothing special.'

'Well then, have the operation over Christmas. It's a disrupted period anyway. And then you can convalesce in the New Year. Agreed?'

'Just a moment,' I said. What was he talking about? Convalesce – just what kind of major operation did he have in mind? I felt as if I had fallen in front of a huge vacuum cleaner which was irresistibly sucking me into its dark innards. Stop pushing me, I thought, what's the hurry? 'Just a moment . . . surely it can't be that urgent?'

'I advise you to have the operation over Christmas,' said Dr Colville in a rich, me-God-you-ignorant-worm tone of voice and clamped his jaws together to show that there would be no more words forthcoming. So I decided to take the bull by the horns and ask the question which my inner voice had suggested a few times in the past.

'Is it melanoma?' I asked casually.

'Of course it's melanoma.' He was stating the obvious, answering a child's silly question. But then his eyebrows shot up. 'How do you know about that? Do you come from a medical background?'

'No, but I was trained as a reporter, and in my job I pick up a great deal of . . . assorted information.' I did not allow his verdict to sink in just then. I could see that he was annoyed with himself for falling into my trap, but he composed himself and leaned back in his chair.

'Have you ever lived in the tropics? Fair-skinned people often get melanoma as a result of too much strong sunshine. In Australia and New Zealand your chances of getting it would be quite high. In Africa, too.'

'I've never been to Australia or New Zealand. And the only time I spent in Africa was ten days in Khartoum where the sky was overcast the whole time and where I popped from one air-conditioned building into the next. Otherwise – surely holidays in Greece in May or September wouldn't qualify as tropical? Besides, I don't sunbathe if I can help it. I find it deadly boring.'

'Well then, in your case we can forget about excessive sunshine. And we don't know what else can cause melanoma. But if it's tackled early, you have nothing to worry about. Let me just check one more thing,' he said, coming over to me. 'Do excuse me if I appear cheeky . . .' Gingerly he lifted my skirt and probed my

27

right groin, a move I found baffling. 'That's fine,' he said, looking down at me from his great height. I had no idea what was going on. 'The pigmented naevum – that's your brown spot – will be removed and you'll have a wide excision done on your right leg – oh, say twenty centimetres by ten. And then you'll be given a skin graft from your left thigh. To cover up the hole, so to speak.'

I gasped. 'But that's an enormous area to remove! Why does it have to be so large?'

'To prevent further trouble. To make sure nothing is left behind that shouldn't be there. If we only removed the bit immediately surrounding the trouble spot, in a few years' time you might get something much worse and you'd be furious with us. Quite rightly, too.'

In my mind's eye I now saw my right leg in the form of a map. The brown spot was the centre of the danger zone which stretched in an irregular manner up north towards the knee and down south towards the ankle, and the whole zone was covered with small, squiggly imaginary lines, indicating the spreading power of . . . of the melanoma, if that's what it was. But how did this polished, ageing man *know* that it was melanoma, after one swift glance? How? Probably by having spent much of his life looking at problems just like mine. In which case he knew just how far no-good cells could travel. That was logical enough. But even so every bit of me – body, mind, feelings, nervous system – felt taut, in the fight-or-flight mode, because Dr Colville was prescribing surgical rape against the integrity of my body, to eliminate a trouble I barely knew I had. I felt cold inside and out, and slightly shell-shocked.

'Do you know a good surgeon?' he asked. 'No? Well, I've got just the man for you. Extremely good at skin grafts, very experienced.' From his desk drawer he fished out a visiting card and handed it to me. 'There you are. Go and make an appointment at once. Mr Lennox's consulting rooms are just round the corner.'

'I'm sorry,' I said, 'I really must get back to my office now. I'll ring Mr Lennox's secretary later.'

'No, I want you to drop in there now. Getting through on the telephone may take longer.'

His insistence irritated me. My personal version of the principle of no taxation without representation demanded that I must not be forced into anything without being given pretty good reasons for it. 'Surely it can't be that urgent,' I said. 'Surely whatever I have can't be so bad that I have to rush into an operation. It's not as if this spot on my leg stopped me from eating or breathing, is it?' He didn't reply. 'Are you saying that if we don't deal with this thing at once, I'm going to die?'

'We are all going to die, dear lady,' he said. 'Seriously, please be sensible and don't put off making your appointment with Mr Lennox. He's a very busy man and may not be able to see you at once.'

'And what about this spot, then?' I asked, pointing to a large, irregular brown patch on my left jaw, next to my ear, which had been bothering me for reasons of vanity. 'Is this also to be removed?'

He ran his fingertips over the patch. 'Goodness, no, that's an ordinary age spot. I always tell my students to watch out for the texture of these things. If they feel velvety, they're harmless age spots. The only trouble with them is that they can't be removed.'

'Not even with special creams?'

'Particularly not with special creams. Once they appear, they're there for life.'

The audience was over. I was glad to say goodbye to Dr Colville, gladder still to leave his rooms in the large building in Harley Street that was a warren of consulting rooms, administrative offices and heaven knew what else. Having lived much of my life with no need for medical treatment, I now felt a lively antipathy for the atmosphere of the bustling medical beehive I had just left. Also, I realised how much I disliked Dr Colville. By his snap diagnosis, which I suspected was wrong, and by his pressing referral for surgery he had changed the flavour of my existence – from healthy to possibly cancerous – and determined my immediate future without making the slightest human contact with me. He had talked at me and through me but not to me, not even for a moment. I felt disturbed and belittled by his divine indifference to me as a person and, perhaps because of my negative feelings towards him, I refused to accept his diagnosis at face value. But what I needed most at that moment was to be comforted, so I went to my favourite café in Wigmore Street, had a coffee with a croissant and butter, smoked a cigarette, and through those basic pleasures quickly reassured myself about my autonomy and freedom of choice.

Even so, reluctantly, I called on Mr Lennox's secretary and made an appointment for the following Friday. Then I hurried towards Oxford Street, away from the Harley Street area, doleful with its doctors and disease. It is a false alarm, I thought, there is nothing to it, but I will follow it through just to prove that I am as healthy as I feel.

The week was busy both at work and in the evenings, but every time I became absorbed enough to forget about that threatening mark on my leg, it promptly popped back into my consciousness. It was like living with a time bomb strapped to my body.

My immediate problem was what to say to Hudie, my love and companion for thirteen years. (I was happily divorced, the way some people are happily married, on friendly terms with my ex-husband, keeping in touch while keeping our distance.) My relationship with Hudie was apparently indestructible. We had had some spectacular ups and downs and several breaks but had always bounced back, sometimes to our mutual astonishment. At first glance we do not look particularly compatible, but we share some vital qualities and needs: needing, for instance, warmth and closeness as much as we need separateness and privacy.

He is grounded, practical and utterly reliable; I tend to get entangled with airy theories and riveting but useless information. He is self-sufficient and solitary; I am gregarious and avid for communication. Unlike me, he is patient, tolerant and forgiving, which may explain why we have lasted so long. What saves him from too much virtue and placidity is a flamboyant, extravagant streak worthy of Louis XIV, and occasional bouts of endearing pig-headed obstinacy.

We had no secrets from each other, but now, faced with an ominous situation, I did not know how much to tell Hudie. As he was a great worrier, I wanted to spare him avoidable anxiety, especially because I knew that any potential threat to me would trigger his fear of separation, loss and death. The subject of death had long been one of our unresolved areas: I knew that it scared him, he knew that it did not scare me. I longed for him to come to grips with his fear yet felt that I must not speak unless he broached the subject. It did not occur to me at the time that sheltering him from a major reality, such as death, was not only foolish but downright patronising. After all, who was I to decide what a grown man could or could not take? But all these considerations were pure theory once more. As my appointment with Mr Lennox was drawing close, I had no option but to tell Hudie what was happening.

He was as astounded by the threat of melanoma as I was myself, but with his unquenchable optimism, which somehow co-exists with his infinite capacity for worry, he decided that the spot would turn out to be harmless. Yes. Well, I hoped so, too, I said, wondering whether we were kidding each other.

Friday came and at midday I was back in Harley Street once more. Mr Lennox seemed strikingly young; not just the way policemen grow more and more youthful as we glide into middle age but absurdly young and slight, with the air of a bright, old-fashioned, short-back-and-sides sixth former. Was he old enough to be a surgeon, let alone an experienced one? But as we shook hands I noticed that in fact he was older than his schoolboyish features suggested: a little lined, dry and tired, and distinctly undernourished. Because he had a shy smile and his suit looked slightly shabby and his stance was gauche – in brief because he looked the exact opposite of the elegant and divinely assured Dr Colville – I immediately took to him.

I told him the story so far. He, too, asked if I had ever lived in the tropics, and confirmed that excessive sunshine was the main identifiable cause of melanoma. 'But then,' he added, 'we don't even know whether you do have melanoma. May I have a look at your leg?'

We went to the examination room next door. I removed my tights and lay down on the couch. Mr Lennox contemplated my right shin. The room was so quiet that every now and then the silence seemed to sizzle for a moment, like oil hitting a hot frying pan. I was beginning to feel hot, too.

'I can't tell what this is without a biopsy,' Mr Lennox said at last. 'It may be perfectly harmless, something like a cyst breaking through. Or else it may be something that has lain dormant for a while and is now becoming active.'

'When you say active, do you mean malignant?' He nodded. 'Please tell me exactly what you mean,' I went on. 'I'm an adult, I'm not afraid and I don't need euphemisms. I'll only feel secure if you tell me the facts as they are.'

'Yes, of course, if that's what you prefer.' He smiled, looking down at me on the couch. 'This thing may be melanoma, as Dr Colville suggested, but without a biopsy we can't know for sure. So I'd like to do the biopsy as soon as possible, and then, *if* we're faced with a malignancy, we'll deal with that immediately. As Dr Colville has no doubt explained to you . . .'

His voice went on, but I let go of it and sat up. The couch had become unpleasantly hot. I realised that it was electrically heated in the already stifling room. But what disturbed me more than the heat was that Mr Lennox was talking down at me from above, standing over my supine body in the classical pose of pagan priest surveying sacrificial victim, parent inspecting baby or magician about to saw the lady in half, and I felt with passion and urgency that that was not the position in which I wished to discuss my future, my chances of health or disease. Did the apparently meek and mild Mr Lennox have an unconscious power complex, was he trying to turn me into a dependent patient when I was still neither?

'Excuse me,' I said, getting off the couch and standing up straight to face him eye to eye. 'This couch is really too hot.' That was the polite coward in me, justifying my rebellion. I did not have the guts to say that I preferred to make decisions standing on my feet rather than lying on my back.

It was then that Mr Lennox first gave me his special look which I was to experience several times in the weeks to come: a level, not unfriendly look of patience mixed with resignation, the gaze of a weary teacher faced with a stupid or troublesome pupil who would have to be subdued before long. 'As I was saying,' he resumed, 'and as Dr Colville told you, you may need a wide excision and a skin graft, with skin taken from your left thigh. Would you mind sitting on that chair for a moment . . .' and he, too, examined my right groin, feeling for heaven knew what. 'That's fine,' he said. 'Can we do the biopsy this afternoon?'

'No, we can't.'

'May I ask why not?'

'Because I'm extremely busy at work.' I found it hard to hide my exasperation. 'I'm working on a script that no one else can finish, it's scheduled for Christmas, it's a commitment I can't break.' My work ethic was furiously beating off the dictates of his. 'And besides, what's the hurry? Why must we rush things? Both you

33

and Dr Colville give the impression that unless we act at once, my life will be in danger. Surely it can't be that urgent?'

There was a long pause. Then he said, 'No, it's not that urgent. But once there's the slightest suspicion of something being not quite right, it's best to act at once. How long do you need to finish your script?'

'My deadline is next Wednesday.'

'That's five days from today – yes, it should be all right.'

He was a reasonable man, I concluded, as he took me to his secretary's room to make arrangements for the biopsy in a West End hospital. It would be done under local anaesthetic, Mr Lennox said, and I would be able to go home under my own steam, but then I would have to stay at home for a few days and put my leg up.

'There's every chance that the biopsy will be the end of your troubles,' he said, seeing me off at the top of the gently curving antique staircase. In that case, I asked, why had Dr Colville been so sure that I was suffering from melanoma? Mr Lennox smiled and shrugged. 'Dr Colville belongs to a generation of doctors who think they're infallible, and of course much of the time they are right. But not always.'

My relief was enormous. Mr Lennox may not have intended to support me against Dr Colville, but that was the effect of his bland comment. He was a nice, reasonable, unpompous man whom I could trust. I rushed into the midday busyness of the world, feeling reassured and optimistic. I was walking very fast, without strain or effort; I had no aches or pains, and every part of my body was functioning well. Surely if I had anything as serious as melanoma, I would feel less fit?

I made the same point two days later, on Advent Sunday, to my friend Catherine, over dinner in South Kensington. She had been my closest friend for a dozen years or more, and I often felt that ever since our first

34

meeting we had been conducting a continuous dialogue, without the slightest hope of ever covering our multitude of shared subjects. Catherine was a psychotherapist, much involved in the training of counsellors. She and her companion John, himself a psychotherapist, also ran a series of highly original workshops on self-discovery (which, I knew from personal experience, acted like a blend of balm and dynamite on a weary psyche). Catherine was small and pretty and as bright-eyed and fearless as a robin. I loved her for her warmth and wisdom and for her finely honed mind that never missed a trick, a nuance or, above all, a meaning; and I cherished just as much her irreverent sense of the absurd and her delicious sense of humour. Catherine was a woman for all seasons, equally interested in bookshops and dress shops, fond of good food and drink, capable of child-like enjoyment. But she also possessed a quality of stillness and depth which I privately thought of as her Himalayan streak: it was present all the time, like a quiet, meditative note sounding behind the bright music.

Over the years we had shared countless meals and bottles of humble wine all over the affordable restaurants of South Kensington. We had talked endlessly about problems both personal and planetary and had laughed a great deal. We had also cursed and sometimes even cried a little into the plonk when things had become too painful.

That evening, on Advent Sunday, I told Catherine what was going on. Like Hudie, like myself, she also took an optimistic view of the biopsy's likely outcome, and only wanted to know how I felt about this strange development. Fine, I said truthfully; in balance, waiting, not afraid, in fact mobbling (which was our word for the way in which a well-made mobile recovers its shape and balance after any disturbance). Besides, I added, I was not the type of personality who was likely to get cancer, was I? Some time before, when I had been working on a radio feature on cancer, she and I had talked a lot about the British and American research into the so-called cancer personality, characterised by emotional repression and the inability to express anger, aggression or love spontaneously.

'You know me inside out,' I said, 'I am not a bit like that, am I?'

'No, you aren't, not now. But remember how long it took you to begin to express your anger. Sometimes I think you're still not sure how to let it out, after repressing it all your life.'

'Since the age of four, to be exact.'

'That's what I had in mind.'

I pulled a rueful face. 'God, it's so vivid. If only I could draw – perhaps drawing the scene would exorcise it. My mother in her beautiful pink silk dressing-gown standing in the bedroom door, absolutely furious, eyes flashing, telling off somebody outside, and I sitting in my little white bed and thinking, I must never lose my temper, I must never get angry like this because it's ugly and dangerous . . . one lot of anger is enough in one family. And how I kept that vow over the years! It's astounding.'

'I'd be happier if I knew that you've finally broken it. I'm not so sure.'

'Oh, but I have. Except you never see me when I let rip.'

Whatever Catherine thought of that, she let it pass. We ate well. The wine was not bad and we toasted the start of Advent, just as we habitually remembered solstices and equinoxes, feasts and festivals whose symbolism felt relevant. On the way home I pondered Advent and saw it as a solitary bright candle floating in unfathomable darkness, utterly alone but unabashed. I could accept that; but what sort of Christmas was it floating towards? Oh, go step by step, cross it when you reach it. At home, alone in my still, sheltering little house I went to sleep at once and did not budge until the morning.

Back at work I finished my script and then told my bosses what was happening. They were concerned but optimistic and strongly supportive. We agreed that for the time being I would – officially – be away with 'flu. If all went well, we would never have to amend that story. Preparing for the biopsy was rather like organising a short business trip, dovetailing small arrangements. Every now and then I listened inwardly, as it were, questioning my body as to whether it was well or ill, running well or running down, but there was no reply except for a general sense of well-being.

It was at that bleak moment in early December, the day before the biopsy, that a clump of April-flowering perennial daisies in my garden suddenly produced a single, perfect, golden-yellow bloom, shaped like a small sun and radiating like one in the winter gloom. It looked heroic and unseasonal, and it made me think of *The Secret of the Golden Flower*, the ancient Chinese text on the quest for spiritual immortality. It was through Jung's commentary on the Taoist text that I first became acquainted with it during one of my periodic immersions in Jung's writings. But the Golden Flower must be a universal archetypal symbol, because I had repeatedly caught glimpses of it in dreams and fantasies, always acting as a saving or redeeming entity, able to light up darkness or lead one out of some deadly maze. Among my personal choice of numinous symbols the Golden Flower came first. And now it was right there, in my small, catatonic garden, surging from a dormant clump of muddy leaves that would hardly stir for another four months.

That flower, I decided, was a good omen.

On the 6th December around noon I presented myself at the small hospital near Leicester Square where Mr Lennox was to perform the biopsy. After a brief bout of administration I ended up in a small room where a chatty nurse asked me to strip down to my underwear. While I changed into paper gown and slippers, she talked glowingly about Mr Lennox. 'Such a wonderful man,' she said. 'We're all happy to work for him, he's always kind and considerate, not like some others, and he never loses his temper. You couldn't be in better hands.' She sounded genuinely enthusiastic, and it did me good to listen to her.

In the small operating theatre Mr Lennox, gowned and capped in bright green, hailed me as if I had arrived at some fun-packed disco party. He looked relaxed, cheerful, almost rakish, a man in his element, exercising his skill and enjoying it. I took a deep breath and lay down on the table.

Throughout the operation we chatted brightly, mainly about broadcasting and favourite programmes. I was in great form, almost manic, entertaining Mr Lennox and the two nurses as if that had been the sole purpose of my presence. As I felt no pain, it was easy to pretend that nothing important was happening, nothing more ominous than tackling an ingrowing toenail. And then it was all over. I was being bandaged, packaged, helped up and allowed to go home. Mr Lennox handed me some painkillers for later use. 'Keep your leg propped up and walk as little as possible,' he warned. 'I'll ring you as soon as I receive the pathologist's report, possibly tomorrow.'

Slightly dazed, I travelled home by underground, wondering what my numb leg looked like within the bandage. At home I made myself comfortable on the long sofa near the telephone, right leg propped up on the sofa's back, a pile of books and fruit within reach. Hudie rang, then Catherine, then my deputy boss. I reassured them and then resumed my silent rest. How odd, I thought, to be at home early on a Wednesday afternoon instead of being at work, when I am not even ill.

The following afternoon around teatime Mr Lennox

rang to say that the spot on my leg had proved to be malignant and that I would have to have the operation. 'I'll try to get you a bed as soon as possible,' he said, mentioning a hospital in Central London where my private group insurance entitled me to a place. 'Please don't worry,' he said in his light, precise voice, 'we'll get rid of the trouble and you'll be as good as new. Have plenty of rest and don't even touch the bandage. I'll ring you about the hospital arrangements within a day or two.'

'How long shall I have to stay in hospital?'

'Oh, between two and three weeks. Depends on how you get on.'

'As long as that?'

'I'm afraid so. But it's a pleasant hospital, with all-day visiting.'

I lay stock still on the sofa. So it was cancer. The carefully balanced inner pattern of the past ten days suddenly shattered, as if a kaleidoscope had been hit with a sledgehammer. I could no longer maintain my mood of non-committal interest, expecting the threat of serious disease to vanish. Now I knew it would not, could not, do that. Even so, I was utterly astonished at the thought of having a malignant process, the worst of all diseases, silently working away inside my apparently healthy body, without producing the smallest symptom. Surely you did not get cancer unless you were debilitated, unwell, suffering from a multitude of symptoms, or perhaps deeply unhappy? Yet I was not any of these things.

I closed my eyes and considered my life, looking for psychosomatic cancer clues and finding none. On the whole I found I was happier than I had been for a long time. My relationship with Hudie was the best and most lasting attachment of my life. My small house near the Thames was my first home that was entirely to my liking, chosen and shaped by me with no interference nor need to compromise. I had exceptional friends whom I looked upon as my family, having no real one; each one chosen, not inflicted by chance, and much loved. I had a good job, stimulating bosses and colleagues and ample responsibility. Sometimes the fiendish commuting and more than full-time pressures felt heavy and irksome and I longed for more freedom and space, yet I could not think of any job I would have preferred. Besides, I was already planning my next career: early retirement, a return to freelance writing, combined with counselling in which I had recently trained. All in all, I thought, this was a good and vigorous pattern, not a negative and miserable one, and I recalled the late Sir Heneage Ogilvy's dictum, 'The happy man doesn't get cancer,' which had so shocked his medical colleagues and which made so much sense if one thought of body and mind as inseparable parts of a whole. None of which helped me. Damn, damn. If I had cancer, then I could not have been really happy, or perhaps Ogilvy's theory was wrong. Or something.

I thought of my mother, my only blood relation. She must not know about this, she would worry herself sick. Mother was eighty-one and lived in a small town on the edge of the Black Forest in West Germany, close to her oldest surviving friend. She had moved there five years before when London had become too exhausting for her. Throughout her ageing, with its gradual losses and growing complaints, I had been the strong, healthy and relatively young one on whom she could rely, and for me to fall ill with cancer at the age when her only health problem had been a slipped disc seemed unforgivable, almost a betrayal of trust. At least that was how I saw it. Somehow or other I had to keep the bad news from her, especially since she was terrified of cancer.

Having reached that decision, I emptied my mind and lay very still, in a state of meditative nothingness. It was the only way I knew to create peace and put a space between myself and the immediate future, the state recommended by Krishna in the Bhagavad Gita:

'Be in peace in pleasure and pain, in gain and in loss, in victory and in the loss of a battle . . .' Had I lost a battle, or was it about to begin?

Later I rang Hudie, Catherine and some other friends who were all waiting for the biopsy result. Malignant – such a showy, evil word, suggesting a villain straight from a melodrama, the kind who stabs people from behind Gothic pillars. Yet I had to use the word to describe my condition, and then I had to cope with the shock, love and concern that rushed at me through the telephone, until it became almost too much.

I also rang my medical herbalist and asked her whether I should have the operation or try some unorthodox therapy instead. 'All I want is an opinion,' I said. 'I'm not asking you to make a decision for me, only I can do that, but what do you think? You've been looking after me for eleven years, you know my general condition pretty well by now . . .'

'Melanoma is a very tricky cancer,' she said after a pause. 'It's totally incalculable. Perhaps the sensible thing is to have the operation and hope that that'll be the end of your troubles. After all, you're pretty healthy.'

Well, that was that. She was right, I thought. Alternative therapies were fine for most things but when it came to a real nasty, it was wiser to stick to established methods. I closed my eyes. The room was warm and very quiet, lost in the darkness of a single-candle Advent. Why did disasters so often strike before Christmas, I wondered. If it is not the boiler that breaks down it is a love affair that breaks up, and if it is neither then you are told that you have cancer and must have an operation over Christmas.

'Be in peace . . .' I got up gingerly and walked to the kitchen window. Even in the darkness outside I could see the solitary golden daisy shining bright in my dead garden.

2

TOWARDS EVENING ON the 12th December Hudie
drove me to the hospital in Bryanston Square. We did
not talk much during the drive. Everything that needed
saying had been said in the past few days and we were
both emotionally drained. The streets looked black and
glistening after a wintry downpour. My leg hurt a little.
That was the only sensation I registered. All else –
thoughts, feelings – had vanished underneath a still,
serene detachment that contained neither fear nor
apprehension; in fact, I was beginning to recognise it as
the phenomenon that had overtaken me several times
in the past, always at a time of acute crisis and danger:
a totally irrational serenity based on the realisation that
all was exactly as it should be and that, however
appalling the current situation seemed, it was all right.
Why was it all right? I did not know. But I sensed that
things were happening in two separate dimensions.
The crisis and danger, the disease and pain belonged to
one dimension, but my consciousness operated in the
other, at least part of the time, and the certainty,
serenity and unshakable sense of rightness of that
second dimension were somehow more real than the
apparently real physical experience. The only thing that
saddened me was that I could not share my mysterious
sense of well-being with Hudie. He would have thought
that I was denying my true feelings.

The hospital did not look like one. It might have been
a block of offices or apartments, with a smart receptionist and a streamlined lobby. Hudie carried in my bag,

hugged and kissed me and rushed out. Neither of us could have borne another moment together. I noticed several shiny ashtrays in the waiting area. Did the permissiveness extend to patients' rooms, too, I wondered, longing for a cigarette.

Sister, called by the receptionist, was middle-aged, unsmiling. 'Don't let them institutionalise you,' my friend Pat had warned me on the telephone that morning. Sister struck me as the sort of person who would at least try to do just that. She was dry and unsociable, disinterested, refusing to make the slightest, most fleeting contact. Up in Room 47, which was bleak and overheated, she entered my particulars in a ledger. Next of kin? I gave Hudie's name. Any drugs? I shook my head. The herbal and homoeopathic remedies, provided by my herbalist to diminish surgical shock and promote healing were not drugs, and I was determined to hang on to them. Religion? RC, I said; should have added 'inactive', in brackets, like RN (retired), but did not. Perhaps for official purposes it was wiser to give one's official religion rather than try to define one's actual unofficial creed, in my case something like free-range Christian with strong Buddhist sympathies and an abiding love for the Bhagavad Gita. Sister would not have liked that.

After her departure I inspected my room and found it dismal, a pretty successful attempt at total sensory deprivation. Walls, paintwork, bed, cupboard and shelves were all dead white. Only the lino and the tubular easy chair struck an equally dead beige note. No pictures on the wall, not a scrap of colour or texture, nothing to deflect the mind from sadness or anxiety. Mercifully the window opened onto the square and the tops of the mighty London plane trees, bare and bold against the sky, filled the entire large window. Immediately I felt less cut off. Trees were among my great loves. They knew how to be well-rooted while reaching towards the sky; even in big cities I had never lived far

43

from trees. Now it was a tremendous relief to see them, and Room 47 needed all the relief it could get.

Dinner arrived on a tray and remained on it, practically intact. It was all dead food: thin tinned soup, thin leathery meat, drowned vegetables, sliced white bread, tinned plastic fruit compote, the kind of detestable food that left one both bloated and hungry. It annoyed me that even this much-praised hospital served food that smacked of a third-rate seaside café, and I decided to organise my own food supply in the morning. There was an ashtray on my bedside table. I knew I should ignore it, but I smoked a cigarette instead and then went out, for a change of scene, to the corridor.

The typed label on my door showed my name and, underneath, that of Mr Lennox. It looked odd, as if we had been sharing a room. The doors of two adjacent rooms were open. In one I saw a heavyweight man sitting up in bed, talking with two visitors. Except for his colour which was nearly as purple as his pyjamas, he seemed in good fettle. But in the other room the patient was alabaster-pale. He was lying stock still on his bed, looking as cold and fragile as a sliver of ice. Was he before or after his operation, indeed was he alive or dead? Across the landing a nurse hurried out of a room and left the door ajar, allowing me to glimpse a dishevelled woman festooned with tubes, face yellow, hair like a bird's nest, an air of grim helplessness around her. The unnatural way in which she held her thin hands made me uneasy. I felt I belonged to another country, being strong and fit and normal except for the bandage on my leg. Was I acting out a real-life version of those awful dreams in which you leave the lift on the wrong landing, the train at the wrong station, and are hopelessly lost for ever? What on earth was I doing there anyway?

'Please be in bed by nine,' said Sister, suddenly materialising by my side. 'You want to get a proper rest.' I nodded. Yes, bed. There was nothing else to do, except perhaps pick up my things, go home, opt out of the system. But the temptation was brief. Besides, I had already signed a form promising to pay all my hospital bills; it was too late to change course. I went to bed, took my herbal and homoeopathic remedies furtively, like a junkie administering a fix, and began to read.

There was a knock on the door and a man entered before I had a chance to reply. His face was as crumpled as his clothes, he looked grey with fatigue and he reeked of stale tobacco. Someone's visitor gone astray, or, more likely, a newly arrived patient steered to the wrong floor, I thought – but no, he turned out to be the anaesthetist come to take my pulse, listen to my chest, make me cough and ask a few questions. It was all over in a few minutes. He was satisifed with my condition, I felt concerned about his. If appearances meant anything, he should have been in a hospital bed, not me.

He left. Minutes later a nurse burst in, bearing sleeping tablets and a dose of laxative. I refused both. But she insisted on feeding me a sleeping tablet, to keep out the traffic noises, as she put it. Double glazing would have been more to the point, I pondered, but I did not want to establish myself right away as a so-called difficult patient, so I swallowed the Mogadon and put the light out. Through the half-open curtains I watched the treetops traced in black against the London night sky which is never quite dark, not even in the dead of winter, and the large criss-crossing branches evoked the whiff of a memory that took me a little while to drag to the fore.

But then I knew. The interlacing branches outside reminded me of the plane tree of Hippocrates on the island of Cos, an ancient giant that is more of a circular grove than a single tree, its massive limbs resting on broken columns and other bits of antique masonry. It is an extraordinary tree that has the powerful presence of a wise and venerable person who has understood the secret of life and has found it endearingly simple.

Hippocrates of Cos was supposed to have taught his students beneath those branches, except that the tree is not old enough for that. But it looks right for the legend. Besides, who knows how a numinous, magical *platanos* renews itself, who knows whether that vast tree that today covers a whole square with its shade had not started as a single shoot rising from the dying trunk of Hippocrates' own tree?

Remembering that tree unleashed a flood of images from my memory bank, all of them connected with Greek healing sanctuaries. I saw the three terraces of the majestic Aesculapion of Cos, and the crystal-clear healing spring flowing eternally from the hillside; I saw the peace and beauty of Epidauros, navel of the world; and then my built-in cinema produced the image of my favourite healing centre, the small, secretive Amphiaraion near Athens, hidden in a deep valley alongside a brook. Ruins, birdsong, dark pines, a carpet of anemones in the spring. Above all the calm, reassuring atmosphere of a place where healing was possible. Lying in my Hi-Tech hospital bed with its multiple levers and pulleys, I was overcome by a longing for a simple, calm form of medicine that treated the whole person, not just an illness. I had often discussed that with friends who worked in various branches of alternative medicine; now, when my need for the alternative approach was really keen, I found myself marooned in the other camp.

To comfort myself, I carefully reconstructed the Amphiaraion behind my closed eyelids, with its small temple and its little theatre open to the sky as well as to catharsis, laughter, tears. There, I fantasised, I would be sleeping in a stone cell, lulled by herbs and by the splashing brook into the state of *incubatio*, and in the morning a healer-priest would listen to my dream which would then serve as diagnosis or even as prescription (as it so often does in psychotherapy) . . . I certainly would not be given a drug that actually inhibits dreaming. And then I slept.

Early next morning, instead of a silent healer-priest, it was a loud-voiced nurse who burst in to wake me. Why does she shout, I wondered, sore and drowsy after my unnatural sleep; why does she implode into my inner space like an enemy? Then I thought, good God, it is my operation today, the 13th December, St Lucy's day, feast of light in the darkness, not a bad day for surgery, or is it? But the nurse was already pumping the pre-med injection into my arm and I soon sank into a deep black soft bottomless vacuum.

I came to on the other shore of the vacuum with two nurses patting my arms and calling me very loudly by my name. My mind cleared fast, but when I tried to ask for water, my speech was so slurred that the nurses did not understand me. Of the operation I had no recollection. My front teeth hurt. Had the anaesthetist knelt on my face? Then other kinds of pain began to register from my toes upward. The heavy bandage on my right leg made movement difficult. But I was not supposed to move anyway. When painkillers were offered, I took them. The hours floated by. Faces floated in and out. Hudie came in briefly, looking anxious, trying to smile but not quite making it. Flowers arrived. I asked Hudie to get me quantities of fruit, black rye bread and plain yoghurt. He went off immediately. I lay there, not quite back in my body, for the unity of body and consciousness had not been restored. The anaesthetic had done something dreadful to me because I could feel my consciousness stuck halfway outside my body, neither free nor rooted; a sensation of being unbuttoned on the deepest level. But then the physical pain and mental discomfort fell silent as a wave of irrational and overwhelming serenity lapped over me. There it was again, the conviction that deep down everything was as it should be, with nothing to grieve or worry about, and I

47

could no more account for that unjustified moment of bliss than I could for my malignant mole.

Mr Lennox appeared, smiling, reassuring. Oh yes, everything had gone well; oh no, he had not found anything alarming. 'We caught it in time, it's all gone, nothing to worry about,' he said. 'I'll do the skin graft in six days' time. It'll take better after that sort of interval. And then you'll be able to concentrate on getting really fit.' As ever, Mr Lennox spoke very clearly, with the crystalline enunciation of an elocution teacher. I concluded that many of his patients must be deaf, dim, or both. Only later did it strike me that Mr Lennox's perfectly modulated diction was, above all, totally impersonal. It held you at arm's length, in a formal mode. Who would, after all, address an emotional statement to a talking clock? But this insight came later. At that moment, in my post-operational twilight, I was glad to hear Mr Lennox's measured tones, glad to learn that he had delivered me from my evil. He said he was sorry about the pain – the nurses would keep me supplied with painkillers.

'What bothers me most,' I said, 'is that I don't know why I got melanoma, and therefore I don't know either what to avoid in future, beside strong sunlight.'

'Well, of course, try to avoid carcinogens; easier said than done these days.'

I was waiting for him to say stop smoking, but he didn't. So I tried another approach. 'Well then, can I do anything to . . . reinforce my defences? What about food, for instance, should I follow a special diet?'

He shook his head. 'Diet has nothing to do with cancer,' he said. 'Just make sure that you eat plenty of good, nourishing food to build up your strength. That's all.'

'Do you realise how abysmal the food is in this hospital?'

'Oh, I've seen worse. And you won't be here all that long.'

Since he had no further advice for me, I began once more to wonder about his diet. Did he have one, did he *eat*, for heaven's sake? A pale, emaciated surgeon and a grey-faced, exhausted anaesthetist make a discouraging team. I wondered what the pathologist looked like. But principally I was concerned with myself, and despite all the vile pain and discomfort I felt glad and grateful. Was it not lucky, I mused, that if I had to get cancer, I should get an easily detectable surface growth, not a sinister, deep-seated tumour that could cause irreversible damage without a single symptom before being discovered. I had got away lightly. With today's marvellous skin graft techniques I might even get away reasonably unmarked.

The next five days merged into a featureless chunk. Days and nights of pain and more pain, being stuck in bed, either propped up or lying flat, either way uncomfortable. The nurses were young and pleasant – German, French, Indian, West Indian, and a tiny, pretty Chinese girl from Hong Kong who was a fountain of smiles. Friends took turns to sit with me. Pat, with her soft Scottish voice and sharp Scottish wit was particularly generous with her time. At last, after twenty-five years of friendship, we almost had enough leisure to discuss all topics of interest. The bedside telephone was a lifeline. I needed contact with the outside world to save me from being completely contained and managed by the system. Not since babyhood had I been so dependent and helpless. It would have been so easy to hand over and regress into passivity.

Hudie came every day, sometimes twice a day, full of anxiety and tension. I tried to reassure him and to inject him with my conviction of the basic rightness of things despite outward appearances, until it struck me as weirdly funny that I should be comforting him instead of the other way round. If I had been afraid, would he have taken over the role of comforter, or would we have been scared together?

My room looked like a cross between a florist's and a fruiterer's, and I ate fruit day and night. I also tried to eat some of the hospital food, provided at such enormous cost, but the meals remained obstinately dreadful and grew increasingly salty. My complaint resulted in a visit by Matron, a stout, heavily made up strawberry blonde in a lilac uniform with matching cap. Scaled down she would have made a good fairy for the top of the tree; full size she was somewhat alarming.

'I heard about your complaint,' she said. 'Do you really find the food too salty?'

If I did not, oh Lilac Fairy, would I have complained? But I only said, 'Yes, I find it quite inedible; more salt than food.'

'How strange,' Matron mused. 'I asked the kitchen two days ago to make the food saltier.'

'What on earth for? You can add salt but you can't remove it. And what about patients with high blood pressure who should be on a saltless diet?'

'Oh?' Matron seemed surprised. 'Very well, I'll tell the kitchen to go slow on the salt. I hope you're otherwise satisfied.'

There was no point in prolonging the conversation, or in wondering why the management did not take nutrition more seriously. The only sensible thing was to eat another two apples.

The lilac Matron was followed by a man in a blue anorak who turned out to be the Padre. He had the sort of kind, anxious face that often goes with bicycle clips and predictable views. At first I did not know who he was, then I did not know why he had come, until at last I realised that he visited all Roman Catholic patients as a matter of routine. We did some conversational figure skating around each other until he asked which church I normally attended for Mass, and I had to admit that I was not a regular churchgoer. This pained him, naturally, and he looked even more bewildered when I told him that I was neither an atheist nor an agnostic but that I preferred to work out my own salvation with diligence.

'Ah, but you can't.' He did not recognise the quotation, and, of course, there was no reason why he should be familiar with the sayings of the Buddha. 'We all need the help of the Church to lead a good life. Isn't this the right moment for you to . . . er . . . review your situation and . . . return to the fold?'

I smiled and said nothing, so he changed direction. 'You may find it difficult to think about these things just now. I daresay you suffered a great deal before you came in here.'

'Oh no, Father. I was fit and well and happy, but all that is being changed rapidly. Once the surgeons get you . . .'

'It may seem like that,' he said earnestly, 'but the surgeons are doing their best and we must get worse before we get better. Of course,' he added, trying yet another approach, 'now you're wondering why God allows us to fall ill and suffer or even die. I must say I find these questions very difficult to answer, so if you're going to ask me why this is happening to you –'

Wrong again, Father, I thought: why do you not ask me first whether I am asking you any questions? I felt some sorrowful affection for the man. He was so bad at his job, so obviously unable to communicate beyond the most basic adult-to-child level. 'You needn't worry about me,' I said, 'I'm not questioning or blaming the Higher Powers for landing me with cancer. I suspect that this illness is happening to me because it's part of my pattern and because I have to learn something that I wouldn't learn otherwise.' Bless the man, I thought with surprise, he has made me formulate a vague inner conviction for the first time; he has helped me by being totally unhelpful. 'There was a woman saint, you know,' I went on, not mentioning that I was thinking of a Muslim mystic of the thirteenth century, 'a woman saint who settled the problem by saying, "All things

51

come to me from Him who is my friend". I rather like that. Don't you?'

Without a word the Padre lurched forward and dropped to his knees. Heavens, I thought, he is over-reacting. Does he take me for a woman saint, too? But no, the Padre was not paying homage to me, he had obviously decided to end our awkward meeting by reciting the Lord's Prayer in the stance of a child, folded hands held high at nose level, the words rattling forth like wooden bullets. I prayed with him. After the amen he jumped up and rushed out of my room.

The nights were the worst. Much of the time the pain in my leg proved stronger than the combined effect of sleeping drugs and painkillers. But when I managed to drop off between two bouts of tortured waking, the dreams came thick and fast. Many of them featured the sea and its creatures. In one dream a talking dolphin appeared, encased in a huge cube of sea water; he asked me to go swimming with him so that he could teach me to dive deep and then leap high up in the air. In another dream I saved a galaxy of brillianty coloured sea crea-tures from the owner of a restaurant who did not realise that they were magical creatures and not the ingredients of a fish soup. My unconscious even invented a flat grey boat that began to glide smoothly on the water as soon as I boarded it, powered by invisible means. Diving, soaring, gliding, the immense freedom of the sea was just what I needed to compensate for the captive and arid nature of my reality.

I could remember only one dream which seemed to comment on my illness and treatment. Its hero was a delightful young man who was my 'other half', my animus figure. I greeted him with joy, and then he was attacked by men in white paper suits and caps – surgeons? – who tore off his right leg and left him lying on the ground. In a rage I attacked the men and found that not only their clothes but their bodies were also made of paper; they were no more than thin, irrelevant cut-outs. I also found that I was able to restore the young man's torn-off leg and make him whole again. Despite that happy outcome the dream left me slightly chilled. I recorded it and then dismissed it from my thoughts.

There were other dreams which no doubt contained relevant messages from me to me, but they were shattered by nurses stampeding into my consciousness at the end of their night-shift. Only the gentle Indian girl wakened me quietly. All the others burst in with the noisy energy of hockey captains, snapping on all the lights, throwing around enough decibels to waken the dead. It hurt, and the ice-cold thermometer felt unpleasant, while trying to wash in bed was a dismal farce. To crown it all, having been wakened, vocally assaulted, fleetingly groomed and propped up in a sitting position, I was abandoned for an hour and more, without breakfast or any other consolation.

Sitting there in the morning darkness, I thought of Dr Leboyer, the pioneer of gentle birth, the first man to champion babies' needs to be born in silence, warmth and soothing semi-darkness, not in the harsh lights and cacophony of hospital delivery rooms. Where was the adults' Dr Leboyer, I wondered, to teach doctors and nurses about allowing a gentle rebirth to hospital patients, especially on the border between sleeping and waking. Why did these nurses only take the temperature of my body but not of my psyche, why did they shock me from one state of consciousness into another? Because they did not even know what the Greeks had known three thousand years ago, I answered to myself, before eating another apple.

Early on the 19th December two nurses put me through the pre-med routine once more. It was skin graft day, when Mr Lennox would transpose a large piece of skin from my left thigh, known as the donor, onto my right shin. But this time the sedation did not work fully. I was dimly aware of being whisked along a corridor on a trolley and even caught a glimpse of the dead-beat anaesthetist in a funny little green cap. 'Oh, it's you again,' I said with a slow, thick tongue. 'Please don't hurt my teeth.' He opened his mouth but I did not hear his answer. Either he or I slipped into a woolly, clouded whiteness, and that is all I remember. Then I was once again back in my room.

Hudie swam into focus. 'All done,' he said, and touched my cheek. I nodded. There were countless little empty spaces in my brain and I was not sure that they would ever close up again. It felt as if some of the wires in my thinking apparatus had been severed, so that I could not make certain connections or responses.

A friend had warned that the donor limb might hurt more than the grafted recipient, and he was right. My left thigh was screamingly sore, aflame, raw and violently painful. Now I knew, at least in part, what it was like to be flayed alive. If a comparatively small flayed area could hurt so infernally, what did a more extensive skinning feel like? Perversely, my memory served up every relevant image I had ever seen, mainly of holy martyrs carrying their flayed skins like as many crumpled cat suits, and a particularly ghastly picture from some small Belgian museum, of black-garbed doctors skinning a greenish corpse. The torment of being parted from a portion of my skin went so deep that I doubted whether I would ever be able to peel an orange again.

Pain, pain. Now both my legs were massively and tightly bandaged from toes to groin; the left one, I gathered, as a precaution against the formation of blood clots. A metal frame at the foot of the bed held up the bedclothes in a square tent shape to keep their weight off my sore legs. I could not move or turn to my side. One day the sweet Chinese nurse, noticing that I was depressed, gave me a comforting pat on my left thigh. She might have just as well poured boiling oil over it. The searing pain was so vile that I burst into tears. The girl became flustered; I had to push her hand away as she was about to give me an even stronger pat of comfort and sympathy – and then explain my brusque gesture.

Mr Lennox dropped in every day, often twice a day. His visits were of a social nature, because for the time being he did not wish to disturb my bandaged parts. 'Let nature do her job,' he said, 'without the dirty hands of surgeons and nurses interfering in the healing process.' Why dirty, I wondered inwardly, did he not wash his hands before examining a patient? But the question remained an inward one. Looking back, I find it significant that our exchanges were consistently humorous, as if we had been rehearsing for a Wit and Wisdom contest. I was acting out the role of the good, courageous patient as I saw it at the time, while Mr Lennox was no doubt pleased to find me co-operative, free from despair and, above all, unemotional. I played his game and he rewarded me with encouraging remarks about my progress and cancer-free future.

On the 21st I spent my undisturbed dawn period contemplating the winter solstice, that perfect prelude to Christmas and even a possible uncommercialised alternative to it; after all, both are about the birth of light out of darkness. In the heavy, pitch-black dawn I closed my eyes to experience the blackness, deadness, stillness and void of night, and then the moment when the slow ascent begins, simply because no further descent is possible. I thought of the cyclical nature of life that imprisons us in a cage of polarities – life-death, good-bad, dark-light, joy-sorrow – and allows us no freedom until we learn to reconcile the opposites, stand at the still point in the centre and find balance. My current trap, the polarity of sickness-health, still had to be puzzled out, and I felt more sure of the theory than the practice. But I knew that I had to experience the dark part of the cycle and not pretend that it was, in fact, light.

I asked Mr Lennox whether I would need any further

treatment. Oh no, he said, he had removed the malignancy completely, there was nothing else to do, no radiation or chemotherapy. But I had to be very careful until my leg healed completely – the skin graft was so fragile that the slightest knock would damage it.

'How long will it take to heal completely?'

'Quite a while, I can't even guess at the moment. But you'll have to be very patient.'

That sounded ominous. A few days later when he first removed the massive bandage to inspect the graft, I shut my eyes. For the time being I felt that my right leg belonged to Mr Lennox, and except for keeping it within the boundaries of my body I did not want to have anything to do with it. The severe pain and presumably ghastly appearance of the leg made me distance myself from it.

'You're quite right not to look,' said Mr Lennox, putting on a fresh dressing. 'To me your leg looks beautiful, but you might think otherwise. I must say your general condition is excellent and you're healing surprisingly well.'

Ah, not for nothing was I taking my illicit herbal and homoeopathic remedies three times a day. But I did not tell him about that. He might have asked me to stop taking them and I did not fancy a confrontation.

On Christmas Eve, in the afternoon, I rang my mother in Germany. I told her brightly that my telephone at home had been out of order for some time and that I was ringing from a hotel. 'That's why I couldn't get through to you,' my mother said in a small broken voice. 'I've been trying to ring to tell you that I'm very ill with 'flu.' I could hear that her words struggled out one by one from a congested chest and she sounded deeply depressed. 'I'm all by myself,' she went on, 'all my neighbours have gone away for Christmas, even my doctor is away, skiing in Switzerland.'

Oh God, total desolation, and I could not help her, could not get on the next plane with Hudie to go across and look after her, and celebrate a portable Christmas for ourselves under the municipal Christmas tree in falling snow. 'But your doctor must have a locum, why don't you call him out?'

Mother proved once more that even *in extremis* she always stuck to her principles. 'I won't be examined by some inexperienced youngster who doesn't know me,' she declared. 'You know how much I dislike change and unfamiliar things.'

The frustrations of a lifetime boiled up in me briefly as I collided – for the thousandth time – with her intransigence. But then I saw the tragi-comical side of my mother's invincible rigidity: she would, I felt sure, chide God in the next world for having created an astounding and constantly changing cosmos. Now, however, she still had to cope with this world. 'Darling,' I said, 'please don't be silly. Call out the locum at once, just to put my mind at ease. You don't want a long and nasty illness, do you?'

After a few more points and counterpoints, pleas and refusals I rang off in distress. All right, I had cancer while she only had 'flu, but she was eighty-one and alone. And then the unholy tangle of feelings that had formed between us over many years, a tangle consisting of love, resentment, caring, guilt, impatience and tenderness and a few more unacknowledged emotions enmeshed me once more, and I wept for the time, so long ago, when she was young and I was a child and we were both healthy and on the ascending curve of life, untouched by the shadow of death.

Later that evening Hudie and I celebrated Christmas Eve over a decorated candle and some fir branches. We had a drink, to lighten the distinctly unfestive occasion. Shortly afterwards my right leg exploded in hot pain, especially around the ankle. 'Ah, yes, of course,' said the nurse who answered my panic call, 'alcohol dilates your blood vessels and that's bound to feel very unpleasant. Weren't you told not to drink?'

So drink was out, too. Outside my door there was much coming and going, voices, laughter. Sister came to announce that on Christmas Day I would be taken in a wheelchair to the main landing to see the tree. But she forgot and I spent Christmas Day in bed, catching only faint tinklings of carols from the distance. Among the scores of cards lining my room, the one that stood out bore the message, 'The Christmas I spent in hospital was one of the nicest I've had.' Dear, thoughtful friend; she could not have been in this hospital.

Christmas dinner was heavily traditional. Hudie, as my authorised guest, sat with his tray laid across the arms of a special feeding seat, resembling a child's high chair. We looked absurd, corralled behind our trays which even provided a funny hat and a cracker each. The whole set-up was absurd, and so we laughed and laughed and left most of the pudding.

Around teatime the Padre dropped in to utter a Christmas blessing. He looked uneasy and refused to stay. After that we did not meet again. But then we had never met at any meaningful level.

Finally, quite late, to round off the day, Catherine and John arrived, bearing gifts and a portable bar – whisky, soda, ice, glasses, nuts, the lot. In deference to my sensitive blood vessels I refused to drink – and felt I had made a major sacrifice. They sat on either side of my bed, so that talking to both of them was like watching tennis on television. They had been to see me before, but now, because it was Christmas Day and they were full of stories and vitality and plans for the New Year, their visit was a massive tonic, an antidote to the false reality of hospital life. After they had left I decided that, considering everything, it had been a reasonable Christmas.

The following morning, a muscular nurse arrived to help me out of bed. I would have fallen down in a heap if she had not caught and held me: my legs had turned to cardboard. The nurse helped me into the easy-chair by the window. Feeling like a massive chunk of pain, I thought it was odd that while my cancer had given me neither pain nor trouble, the treatment was inflicting both in vile abundance. I mentioned this to Mr Lennox when he dropped in on his daily rounds. He smiled and asked me if I knew the difference between a medical and a surgical case. I did not? Well, if you were very ill when you came to hospital and they made you better, you were a medical case, but if you arrived in good health and they made you very ill, you were surgical. That sounded roughly right, and I liked him for telling a joke against his profession. Only later did I realise that yet another serious matter had been reduced to a joke.

Mr Lennox said I could go home in two days' time, provided I had a resident helper. Hudie immediately volunteered to move in. I was deeply grateful for that – going home had suddenly become urgent. Mr Lennox spelled out his terms. I was not to go out or do housework until told otherwise. Above all, I was to guard my skin graft against injury as if it were frail china. For a while, he added, I would not be able to put any weight on my right leg and the pain would persevere. But he would drop in regularly to keep an eye on me and change my dressings.

My last night in hospital was the worst. On top of the usual burning pain I felt as if a vice had been clamped on my right ankle and then tightened more and more, until I wanted to tear my leg off. The night nurse was sour, ageing and cold, the first unpleasant nurse to cross my path in three weeks. She tried to be bossy, but when she ordered me to stop fussing, my patience snapped.

'If you can't tell the difference between fussing and suffering great pain, you shouldn't be a nurse,' I told her. 'Please loosen the bandage on my right ankle, or if you have no authority to do that, ring my surgeon and ask for instructions. I can't bear the pressure any longer.'

After some resistance she went off to telephone, came back and snipped open the bottom edge of the bandage. 'That's all Mr Lennox will allow,' she said.

'But the pressure is still terrible, almost as bad as before!'

'Then the tightness isn't caused by the bandage. What's so tight is the skin graft itself, and you'd better get used to that, because it won't improve. Ask Mr Lennox, if you don't believe me.'

What rubbish, I thought; nasty sadistic woman, trying to scare me. Between bouts of flimsy sleep I watched the treetops of Bryanston Square for the last time. They were the only things I was sorry to leave behind.

The next morning I crashed headlong into my total helplessness. I longed to fly but my body could not move at all; a wheelchair was needed to take me to the lift and then to the car where Hudie was waiting. A porter and the ebullient Jamaican nurse, whose life's ambition was to be stuck in a lift with Robert Redford, somehow inserted me in the car, laying me across the back seat. God, how was I going to cope, away from the white womb of the hospital? Hudie drove slowly and with great care, yet I found the outside world, flashing past the car windows, horribly fast-moving and aggressive. In brief, I was scared.

At last we were in my familiar road with its Victorian workmen's cottages and three magnificent lime trees. Hudie helped me to crawl out of the car and into my house. Never had I longed more for levitation; never had I been clumsier, with only my left leg and the hospital-issue metal walking stick to support me. My two lots of pain – burning rawness in my left thigh, sharp twisting pressure in my right leg – began to recede behind a wave of indignation. How the hell did they – Mr Lennox, the hospital, the whole medical hierarchy – expect me to cope with this handicap? I lay down on the sofa and beyond my pain and weariness tried to recapture that earlier serene certainty that all was exactly as it should be. But now I only recovered a faint whiff of it. I knew it was still valid, but it had become almost inaccessible, as if the intensely physical happenings of the past few days had blocked the door to my inner resources.

'You won't believe this,' Hudie called from the kitchen, 'but your golden daisy is still blooming and it's in perfect condition!'

That was how my convalescence began, with total dependence and near immobility. I could only move up and down the stairs seated on my bottom and it took all my will power to make me shuffle across the shortest distance. It was as if I had suddenly grown very old, my body struck by some instant geriatric transformation, while the rest of me remained my normal age, indignant and bewildered. For the first time in my life my body was running the show or, rather, running down and paralysing it, with mind lingering distinctly below matter.

Hudie was endlessly helpful and caring. Somehow he managed to fit in his nursing and housekeeping chores with his work, and he fed and tended me with touching thoughtfulness. He was the male equivalent of a good mother, without the huge drawbacks of the latter. But after a few days the strain of the situation began to tell on us. My constant pain and helplessness made me snappy and touchy. I felt like a twitching bundle of raw nerve endings exposed to a sandstorm; I had even lost the ability to laugh at myself. Hudie, in turn, suffered from seeing me so weak and disconsolate. To him I had always been strong, self-reliant and able to solve problems, and the pathetic change in me threatened his own sense of security. So we had several tense and miserable evenings when I resented everything he said and most things he did. I was also deeply

61

grateful for his help, but the love and appreciation somehow vanished beneath our tension and mutual resentment. In the daytime, when I had time to myself between visitors, I often felt disturbed by my behaviour to Hudie and, beyond that, by the way in which physical suffering had cancelled out my inner discipline and rules of conduct. I saw this clearly and did not like what I saw. It did not fit in with my familiar self-image which was full of flaws but was also, on the whole, balanced, considerate and detached in the face of difficulties. Where had this cantankerous, weak and unreasonable creature suddenly come from? It felt as if my self had been invaded by an undesirable alien. It did not occur to me that perhaps my self-image needed adjusting.

Mr Lennox visited me once or twice a week, always late in the evening, on his way home. He changed the dressings on both my legs, listened to my complaints, made me walk, gave advice and departed. Officially I still refused to look at my skin graft, but once, while he was preparing the fresh dressing, I risked a quick glance through half-closed eyes. What I glimpsed was a raw, dreadful and literally bloody mess, more like something off the butcher's slab than part of my own body. I was too shocked to utter a sound, but at that precise moment Mr Lennox observed in his slow and clear diction, 'This is coming on really nicely, I'm very pleased with it.' Bending low over my dreadful wound, he could not see my appalled face and went on cheerfully, 'Tomorrow you can start going out. Walk a few steps outside the house and then do a little more every day.'

'But I can't get my right foot into any shoe! Why is it so swollen?'

'Because I had to remove some lymph glands and now the lymph can't circulate. It'll take quite a few months for it to find another path, I'm afraid, and until then your foot will be swollen. Don't you have some old shoes that would stretch sufficiently?'

A flayed thigh, a butcher's-meat leg *and* a swollen foot – just how many more ghastly side effects was Mr Lennox's treatment going to bring? Yet I was disarmed by his obvious dedication in coming to change my dressings himself, instead of sending a nurse. So I did not grumble, but borrowed a pair of huge Eskimo-style snow-shoes from a friend, put them on and struggled out of the house. God, did my leg hurt. After five yards I turned back, racked by pain and despair.

But the next day I forced myself to cover ten yards. And then twenty, slowly and achingly, leaning on my stick, dreading a fall. Neighbours who had known me in my speedy days stopped to encourage or commiserate. Eventually, I made it to the street corner and beyond; finally to the river which now seemed fantastically lovely – radiant, glittering, raucous with gulls, ducks and a pair of Canada geese, eternally on the move. Every day I met several other slow-moving women with hospital-issue metal sticks just like mine, but they were very old and very fat and they looked at me as if I was a confidence trickster, far too young and fit-looking to crawl along in such a tormented fashion. Clearly I did not belong to their community and they did not return my smile.

But there was something else to the experience, too.

During those awful weeks when I could only limp along with a stick, I was astonished by the number of crippled, lame and otherwise handicapped people whom I met daily in the small area I could cover. They must have been around all along, only I had not noticed them before. Then I remembered the time, a year or two before, when I had briefly worn a wig, largely for fun: then, too, I had suddenly become aware of scores of other wig-wearers, men and women, going about their business in central London with their artistic hair substitutes as they had done, no doubt, long before my own perception had become wig-sensitive.

No, there was nothing like shared experience to

widen one's awareness. Perhaps, I thought, one day when I move a fraction closer to enlightenment, I will notice that the world is full of Buddhas.

But meanwhile I had other chores. To take over more and more of the household duties from Hudie. To write chatty letters to my mother, now happily recovered, as if I were fit and at work. Eventually, on Mr Lennox's instructions, to travel by public transport. Oh God, the horror of boarding a bus or train with an eggshell china leg that would not bend at the ankle but shot angry forked lightnings of pain in all directions; of being slower and clumsier than anybody else; of getting out of the Underground train at Leicester Square and stopping, paralysed, at the bottom of the escalators that were zipping upwards at an impossible speed. I understood what it must be like to be the weakest and sickliest member of a herd of deer, always lagging behind and falling over until a lion puts it out of its misery. And I knew that I would never again be impatient, as I used to be, with the slow, the clumsy and the helpless.

I had two consecutive dreams which seemed to convey the same message. In one I was trying to cook a whole chicken in the very small saucepan which I normally use for boiling one or two eggs. The bird looked miserably cramped and refused to cook properly. In the second dream a beautiful large fish, a sea trout, was thrashing around in my yellow plastic washing-up bowl and eventually leaped out of it. I put it back but the fish jumped out again, and I realised that it was trying to commit suicide rather than endure the shallow confinement of the bowl. Too little space, not enough freedom, I thought, concluding that my dreams were comments on my current lifestyle.

The following day Mr Lennox declared that in mid-February I could go back to work.

3

THE NEXT FEW weeks smacked of anticlimax. I felt like the stupid woodcutter in the folk tale who was allowed three wishes by a good fairy and realised too late that he had asked for the wrong things. If only I could walk again, go back to work and lead a normal life once more – those had been my wishes, but although they had now been fulfilled, everything remained suffused with greyness. Nothing looked, felt or tasted right, nothing brought joy or even contentment. Energy had to be whipped up through an act of will and ran out quickly. Concentration was still patchy. Often my memory seized up over some commonplace word or I froze in the middle of a sentence because what I had planned to say had slipped down some black hole. I complained about this to John who recalled his own experience with surgery and told me not to worry: the effects of two general anaesthetics within five days were bound to linger on. He felt sure that my brain damage was not irreversible.

The physical pain was easing up. My left thigh, the donor, had grown a new layer of hypersensitive skin. It was striped pink and red, as if it had been branded with a red-hot giant steel comb. The skin graft itself remained purplish-red and uneven, pocked with marks and scabs, so ugly and messy that I suffered a shock of revulsion every time I saw it. But it had largely healed and only needed a crepe bandage for protection. That was progress. Yet I did not feel at ease with my right leg. I did not even feel that it was mine, somehow, because often it behaved capriciously, as if it had been independent from the rest of my body. I would be walking along quite smoothly when suddenly my ankle would be grabbed, or so it felt, and pressed cruelly hard, so that I would look down in alarm to see what was going on. These fits of vice-like pressure were so frightening that once or twice I half expected to see a sinister steely hand squeezing my ankle, a hand shooting up from the underworld or from between the floorboards, in the manner of childhood nightmares, to claim the leg that was not really mine any more.

I mentioned these incidents – without the fantasy of the steely hand – to Mr Lennox when I next went to see him for a check-up, but all he could recommend was patience. He also thought I should wear support hose, the very name of which made me squirm. I did try a pair, though, but all that happened was that the pressure on my leg grew worse. Our increasingly spaced out meetings were pleasant and chatty. I was anxious to prove that I was doing well, progressing nicely and obeying all the rules; Mr Lennox rewarded me with generous doses of approval and reassurance. He still looked pale and undernourished and still wore the same shabby suit in which he had first received me.

What struck me most about our meetings was the loving admiration with which he gazed at the skin graft. It was the look of the proud craftsman contemplating a successful piece of work that pleased the eye and fulfilled a function. My mother used to gaze like that at a newly finished lampshade or piece of fine embroidery at the height of her skills as a needlewoman, which was right and appropriate. But what bothered me about Mr Lennox was that he never examined or even looked at the rest of me, as if my entire body had been an incidental appendage to his lovely skin graft. Except that I did not find it lovely, and one day, sitting up on the examination couch, I said so, too.

'It's so terribly messy and inflamed. When will it settle down and look more civilised?'

'Oh, it's going to improve, but only very slowly. It may take a year or more.'

'As long as that? How appalling. And look, my right leg is now much thinner than the left – I expect it'll flesh out in time?'

Mr Lennox paused before answering. 'No, I'm afraid it won't. It can't. I had to take away quite a bit of flesh and pull the graft really tight towards the back, and so, you see, the leg can't go back to its original shape. Unfortunately.'

My eyes filled with tears. I felt the shock of betrayal. Nobody had told me that beside the hideousness of the graft there would also be so much mutilation, for no very good reason as far as I could see. After all, the side of my leg which Mr Lennox had sliced off had been at a considerable distance from my malignant spot. Had he really had to cut away so much and so deeply? I took some deep breaths to steady my feelings, but all that happened was that the tears rolled down my face and Mr Lennox stepped back from the couch, as if trying to avoid emotional contamination. I looked at my poor right leg, so stick-like and hideous, and I was overcome by misery.

'I'm sorry this is such a shock to you.' Mr Lennox sounded reproachful. 'I thought you realised that a wide excision was bound to leave a mark.' I could see that my grief over a non-medical matter annoyed him, and I remembered similar insensitive reactions from male doctors in the past over much smaller problems. All those medical men were unable to understand, I reflected while wiping my eyes, that a woman could be almost as attached to her body's integrity as to her survival, and that this was not a matter of vanity but something much deeper, tied up with the importance of being as a function. Was he capable of more sympathy, I wondered, if a woman patient grieved over a lost breast or a destroyed face?

'When I became middle-aged,' I told him in an unsteady voice, 'I consoled myself with the thought that come what may, I'd still have good legs – after all, legs last much longer than faces. But now even that comfort is gone. So, you see – '

'Ah, but you're alive and getting better. Isn't that more important? People won't notice that your right leg is a bit thinner than the left. You can always wear textured stockings or boots. Many women now wear boots almost all the year round, don't they?'

I nodded. As Mr Lennox was unlikely to take any interest in women's leggings unless for professional reasons, I assumed that he had had similar conversations with other distressed patients. There was nothing else to say. At least for the time being my disfigurement remained hidden underneath my elastic bandage, and I was not prepared to think beyond that stage.

At work I was given every possible help: light duties, permission to start late and leave early in order to avoid rush hour travel, and constant reminders not to overdo things. So much kindness and caring moved me. For the first time in my adult life I was learning to accept help instead of keeping my flag of self-reliance nailed to the mast. But at another level the universal greyness had seeped into my work, too, until everything I did seemed lifeless and futile. Words had no resonance, fell flat, left no echo. All the subjects I had to tackle seemed oddly identical and interchangeable, and knowing that the dullness lay within me, not in the subjects, did not help.

Things were not going too well with Hudie, either. Now that I had recovered he saw no reason why we should not return to the way we used to enjoy our leisure together, spending weekends in my house in a state of peaceful domesticity. But that was the one thing I was unable to do. It was as if what had nurtured and satisfied me in the past had become unpalatable, yet I did not know what I was hungering for. I thought I needed action, outings, people, more stimulus, less placidity. A certain tension was building up over our differing needs; the only answer seemed to be to spend less time together.

'Nothing is going well,' I complained to Catherine one evening over dinner. 'I don't feel at home in my life, it doesn't fit any more. What the hell's going on? Surely not a second mid-life crisis? I had a big one at forty, it did just about everything a good mid-lifer is supposed to do, so I hardly need another. But it's a crisis all right, and I'm not handling it well.'

'You've been through a pretty rough patch, and you returned to your old way of life without a break, straight from convalescence. How do you expect to feel happy and well?'

'That's true. But it's not just that, it's worse. You see, when things were really grim, I was sustained by a great underlying feeling of . . . I suppose love and trust and peace. And now when things are much better I'm really low and can't recapture that feeling. It's as if someone had removed my middle. I think I need help.'

'I've been wondering why you were carrying your pile without any help,' Catherine said mildly. 'What do you have in mind? Analysis?'

'Oh no. Counselling. I know you can't take me on, we're too close for that, but what about John? Would you please ask him whether he has a space for me?'

John did. I was delighted. He was a good friend, yet not too close for a spell of counselling, and in my battered state I did not feel like taking my burdens to a stranger. Besides, John was unusually perceptive and intuitive; I knew he would detect any attempt of mine to evade sore points long before I detected it. In brief, I liked and trusted him. When I rang him for my first appointment, I felt I was clearing a hurdle: at last I was asking for psychological help and support, acknowledging my need, instead of pretending to be self-sufficient. All my life, I reflected, I had been 'all right', able to cope, well-organised and strong, happy to give but reluctant to accept help. To give, I had often thought, was not only more blessed but also a damn sight easier than to receive. But now that attitude of mine was no more convincing than the chest-thumping of a puny gorilla. At any rate, when I arrived in John's counselling room, which was as large and comfortable as he himself, I felt like a dead-tired weight-lifter about to drop a ton of lead. John, inhabiting one of his huge pullovers and occasionally scattering his notes all around his chair, was a safe harbour; not only because at workshops and through his meditation course I had learnt his language, both in words and in imagery, but because he had the ability to understand and empathise with current pain and suffering – and at the same time to put it into another, higher perspective that promptly and subtly changed the meaning of the experience. Yet despite all this built-in advantage I found it difficult to explain to him why I was there, in need of help.

'It's like slowly drowning in frustration,' I said. 'I feel that I'm not occupying my rightful place in life. Sorry if that sounds somewhat pompous, but that's the only way I can put it. Rightful place. As long as you don't ask me what my rightful place would be, because I've no idea, except that it's not where I'm now.'

'All right. Where are you now?' When I did not reply, he smiled, pulled a face that suggested 'You know what I'm going to say next,' and then said it: 'Can you get an image for your present situation?'

The inner picture appeared as soon as he had asked the question. 'Oh yes, it's an image from an Indian parable that I read some years ago. It's about a poor beggar who's sitting by the roadside on his shabby mat day by day, year by year, begging. He doesn't get a lot of alms but he still dreams of becoming rich one day and leading a better life. In due course, he dies by the roadside, as poor as ever, and after he's been cremated, the villagers burn his mat and dig up the earth where

70

he used to sit. And two feet down they find a king's ransom in gold, a hundred times more than the beggar would have needed to realise his dream.'

'And you're identifying with that beggar? In that case we'd better go more deeply into that image. Can you see it in full detail?'

I could, in a way that only those who are familiar with imaging can understand. The image appeared inside my closed eyelids with lightning speed and clarity, yet, unlike a picture on a television screen, it was sensed rather than seen. What I perceived at that instant was the image of a dusty roadside in a flat, lifeless landscape that reminded me of the outskirts of Khartoum, to me the ultimate place of desolation and exile. My unconscious choice of location shocked me. Was that what I really felt about my situation, could it really be that bad? The beggar was there, first as a half-naked, dark-skinned man, the archetypal exotic mendicant; then he faded and I saw myself in his place, holding my hand out, waiting. 'Hardly anybody comes this way,' I reported to John. 'And those who come only throw very small coins.'

'Should the beggar move somewhere else?' he asked quietly.

No, no, the point was – why be a beggar at all? I recalled the beggar's image with the ease of rerunning a film, then I returned to my own, and I saw that neither he nor I was crippled or incapacitated; there was no reason why I should not get up, get going and take over the running of my life, instead of waiting for my sustenance to come from outside in the form of small, mean alms. As I kept the image of my begging self steady in the tiny yet infinite space behind my eyelids, I could also see the king's ransom in gold, about a foot and a half deep in the earth beneath the mat; a lovely, gleaming, glowing pile of gold.

'The treasure's all there, right underneath the mat,' I informed John. 'I'll have to go down for it, way below the surface, instead of . . . begging in the dust.' To dive deep – but that is what the dolphin I had dreamt about in hospital wanted to teach me. Perhaps I did spend too much time on the surface, too tied up with my mind.

'How far down is the gold?' John asked.

'Oh, about a foot and a half.' I paused, struck by one of those uncannily accurate 'coincidences' that make imaging so rewarding. 'Do you know, John,' I said in amazement, 'that's the same as the distance between my brain and my heart. Have I been operating on the wrong level all along?'

I returned to my imaginary landscape, taking the beggar's place on the mat. In that instant, a brown door appeared complete with its frame, supported by invisible means a few inches above ground level, right in front of me. I described it to John, noting – with the observer part of my consciousness – that a door symbolised a transition from one state of being to another.

'Would you like to open the door?' he asked.

'No, I'd rather not.'

'Why not?'

'Because if I push it open with my forehead, it'll swing back and bang me on the head. But then – this is crazy. Why on earth should I want to open the door with my head? Am I turning everything into an intellectual exercise? Is that why I'm sitting on the gold, without even knowing that it's there?'

'Well, is it?' And we both laughed.

That is how it started. For the next few weeks I saw John regularly. The detached, exploratory mood of the first session did not last. As we went on, I experienced a great deal of unacknowledged pain and grief from my past, pain that erupted with bitter force. Well, of course, diving deep carried penalties; probably that is why I had been avoiding it with such clear-eyed determination. But John with his warmth and humour and needle-sharp, no-nonsense intelligence provided just the right

sort of security in which to dig up some of the unfinished business and denied pain of my past. Losses,
disappointments, betrayals, broken hopes, missed
opportunities which at the time I had discounted and
dismissed now returned from the dead, larger than life,
demanding to be acknowledged and felt – above all felt
and experienced. After so many dry-eyed years I was
astounded by the volume of tears that wanted to come
out. John sat by, listening in silence or asking the right
question at the right moment, providing paper tissues
and infinite support, and I loved him for it. That early
decision I had made at the age of four, not to lose my
temper nor ever to show anger, must have misfired
badly if it had led to such a complete cut-off of all my
negative feelings that now I found myself – a middle-
aged Alice in a grim Wonderland – swimming around
in a lake of tears.

'Going through all this stuff is like peeling an onion
that grows larger instead of shrinking,' I said to John
one day. It was spring, with the scent of flowering
shrubs wafting in through the window. 'Do you ever
reach the core of the onion? During my counselling
training I worked through so much stuff, I could have
sworn I was in touch with my unconscious material,
but look what's coming up now. Untouched by hand
for twenty-five years or more.'

'I don't think you ever reach the core of the onion,'
John said. 'Not in the normal course of events. But you
can move a fair distance towards it. It all depends on
how far you want to delve.'

I was not sure. Part of me wanted to go on delving,
to weep until the tears ran out, discover what was valid
and what was false in my life and discard the obsolete
and inappropriate ballast. But another part of me knew
that to do so would demolish much of my lifestyle and
demand drastic changes in my work, values and relationships. Did I want that, could I cope with such a
major upheaval?

Something in me decided that the delving had to stop. It was not a conscious decision. I only recognise it now as I contemplate its effects. At any rate when John and Catherine went on holiday, we interrupted our sessions, and after their return I somehow – somehow? – did not resume them. I persuaded myself that the insights I had gained through working with John needed assimilating before we resumed our meetings. Those insights remained with me; in fact, they enabled me to carry on, adapt and adjust. And because I made the wrong choice, adapting and adjusting instead of blowing the false ceiling sky-high, the only thing that gradually changed was the quality of my despair – it was becoming quieter and more manageable, reasonable almost.

I now knew that I had strong unfulfilled ambitions, that by not writing I was blocking whatever creativity I possessed, that my deepening frustration and lethargy were largely self-made; that, indeed, wherever I tried to place the blame for not occupying my rightful place in life, there was no culprit except myself. Now I knew all this, and it made me uncomfortable. If I was really responsible for so many of my problems, could I also be responsible for all of them, directly or indirectly, and, if so, would I be forced to act? Maybe so, but not just yet. First I had to get well, get back to full strength.

Somewhere around that time I decided to eat fish and meat again, after eight successful years as a lacto-vegetarian. I imagined that my body was clamouring for something, and giving it animal protein seemed a sensible measure. Except that it did not stop my vague hankering. For what? I did not know. But I remembered the fasting champion in one of Kafka's short stories who breaks all records and fasts unto death, not because he wants to but because nobody offers him the food he is hungering for.

That summer the dreadful sick headaches that had been troubling me on and off for years became worse and more frequent. They were heavy, migraine-type attacks accompanied by nausea and an overwhelming need for sleep, and they lasted for the best part of the day, stopping me from eating. In the past they had normally followed jolly evenings out with Hudie whose capacity for drink was as generous as his hospitality; once or twice they had been brought on by small amounts of chocolate. But now they came even after a few glasses of light red wine, drunk slowly with a meal. 'It's galloping old age,' I complained to Catherine, 'or else I've become allergic to wine, but whatever it is, I can't bear many more of these headaches. I'll have to switch to beer or mineral water.' Catherine found that possibility appalling. We both regarded wine as an essential part of civilised living; would I have to opt out of that pleasure? For the time being I compromised by cutting down on my intake even more. It did not occur to me that my fits of ghastly malaise might be distress signals from my liver and should be urgently decoded. After all, headaches apart, I was fine.

Except for a series of dental abscesses that plagued me throughout the summer. I had suffered from them for some years; now they, too, were growing more frequent. My dentist, who knew that I hated antibiotics, prescribed them only as a last resort, and he talked sorrowfully about the receding gums of middle-age, and about the pockets that gathered debris until an infection brought on an abscess. It was melancholy stuff. Once again it did not occur to me that, middle-age or no middle-age, so many toxic episodes in quick succession might be a danger signal pointing way beyond teeth and gums. In my tidy way I thought of the parts of the body under separate headings, so that teeth, liver, head and skin graft on the site of a cancer did not hang together, except by courtesy of my all-containing skin.

At the end of June, when I visited Mr Lennox for a routine check-up, he was delighted with the state of my leg. 'Please keep wearing your bandage, though, until that bit in the middle heals and the scab falls off,' he said. 'It's a most vulnerable part and must be protected. How are you otherwise?'

'So-so. I get terribly tired sometimes, to the point of feeling quite stupid with fatigue. It's the worst kind of exhaustion I've ever felt. All my energy just evaporates.'

'So you're overworking again. Why don't you have some early nights? You probably need more sleep than you think. Also, I hope you'll be going on holiday soon – this year you really need a proper break.'

Oh God, he was not listening, did not understand that I was complaining about an unusual kind of tired-ness that was persisting despite early nights – might just as well give up. Whatever I said, Mr Lennox remained convinced that I was in prime condition. There was no need for further visits until the end of the year, he said, and would I ring him in early December for an appointment.

'But that's five months from now!'

'Well, of course, if anything worries you, you must ring me at once. But if all goes well, December will be soon enough.'

Great, I thought, trotting down Harley Street in a brighter mood. Lennox was a conscientious man, utterly dedicated; if he thought I was all right, there was no need to worry about anything.

In September Hudie and I went to France for a fortnight. Our tensions had dissolved and we were once again able to share things in close harmony. Now that I was well again, he did not have to be on constant alert, worrying about my survival, and I was not made cantankerous by pain and discomfort. As usual, we stuck to quiet country lanes as we drove through the Loire and Dordogne valleys to the Auvergne, and we stayed at remote hotels where the only night sounds were owl calls or the chattering of streams. We spent three nights at an isolated hotel overlooking a large lake ringed with lush hills, a place of great healing calm. On the first morning I stood at the window, contemplating the still water of the lake. There were swallows scissoring around the eaves, the sun was a white glow behind the morning mists, and the bells of invisible cows grazing across the water jingled softly. At that moment my dragging tiredness suddenly melted away and I was flooded with a sense of pure joy, as if coming out of a deep depression and finding that the world was incredibly beautiful and as bright as a rainbow. Once again, for the first time in six months, life felt good, right and promising; I had been reborn.

That refreshed, renewed mood stayed on after our return home. I saw Catherine regularly and John occasionally but did not resume therapy with him. The status quo seemed sufficient for the time being; moreover it was pretty similar to the way I had lived before my illness, and that, I thought, was quite an achievement.

Some time in the autumn I came across *A Way To Die*, Rosemary and Victor Zorza's newly published book about their twenty-five-year-old daughter, Jane, who developed melanoma and died of it five months later. After three operations, chemotherapy and endless, dreadful pain and suffering Jane eventually found peace and a dignified death at a hospice, one of a growing number of nursing homes where the highly trained staff use special techniques and much loving care to help the dying. The book, which I found deeply moving and harrowing, was both a memorial to Jane and a plea for extending the hospice movement. I read it with horrified fascination and pity. That poor, poor girl, I thought, less than half my age when she died after so much physical and mental suffering. Clearly, her melanoma had been a different type from mine, more severe, resistant to treatment. Also, I knew, in a young victim cancer spread faster. Jane's disease had started with an ugly dark mole on her right foot, it spread to her right groin, then to her abdomen, then to her bone marrow, by which time nothing could be done for her. (It did not occur to me that even in the earlier stages, when doctors had decided on more surgery or treatment for Jane, they had been unable to influence the progress of her cancer.)

I mourned for Jane as if she had been a close friend, and I felt that if the first operation on her foot had been more drastic, like mine had been, she might have survived. For the first time I was able to look at my mutilated leg without feeling that Mr Lennox had been too scalpel-happy. What depressed me most was the book's all-pervading mood of medical helplessness in the face of cancer in general and of melanoma in particular. Survival seemed to be a matter of luck. And I considered myself very lucky.

When a national newspaper published excerpts from the book, some readers objected, on the grounds that Jane's tragic story was bound to frighten patients suffering or recovering from melanoma. Well, yes, I could see that. If I had not known for sure that I was cured, I might have felt disturbed, too.

4

SUDDENLY IT WAS December. The less there was left of the year, the livelier it became. Once again I felt at home in the world, able to enjoy whatever I was doing. In a vague way I felt renewed, more in touch, free from the sense of bleak isolation that had often hit me in the past few months. My new-found confidence and appetite for life were growing day by day. I felt in great form when I paid a weekend visit to my mother in Germany. She looked well, if a little shrunken, and we talked a great deal, mainly about the past, which was her favoured area, while my antennae were tuned to the future. Even so, it was a good meeting and I left her reluctantly after three days.

Back in London I made my appointment with Mr Lennox for my first check-up since June. It happened to be a fine morning on the 12th December, exactly a year after my operation, and I almost waltzed down Bond Street, full of high spirits. I enjoyed looking at the luxury shops along the street, full of beautiful and totally unnecessary things, silly knick-knacks which nevertheless made a change from the things I normally saw on a weekday morning. With my workload I could no longer go window-shopping, not even at lunchtime, unless I had a very good excuse for strolling in Mayfair, such as visiting my surgeon. 'My surgeon' – it sounded odd; as if no well-appointed household were complete without one. Yet it felt right to think of Mr Lennox as *my* surgeon. We had been through a lot of things together, he had never failed me, and within the strict limits of our professional relationship he was almost a friend. Perhaps, I thought, he will discharge me now.

'Well, I must say, things are a great deal better than they were a year ago,' he said with a thin smile as I lay down on the examination couch. 'You look well. You've lost that tired look.'

'I feel fine. Most of the time. And I can walk quite fast now, almost as fast as before the operation, but I can't keep it up for very long. My right foot still gets swollen below the skin graft; it swells up every after-noon and then it's really painful.'

'That's because the lymph hasn't re-routed itself yet, to make up for the glands which I had to remove. I told you that would take a long time.'

'And the other thing is that I can't drive. My right ankle is still very stiff and it hurts every time I flex it. If I tried to drive, it would probably seize up after a few minutes.'

'It probably would. You'll have to be patient a little longer.' Once again he was contemplating the skin graft with obvious satisfaction. 'This looks greatly improved. But that large scab in the middle does not want to shift, does it? Still, it will, it will, when the wound underneath has healed. The blood supply is poor there, right on the shinbone; that is why healing is so slow. You know, I admire you for not picking off that scab. I don't think I would have enough self-control to leave it alone.'

'I stopped picking scabs off my legs when I was ten.'

'Well, I suppose boys mature much later. If ever,' said Mr Lennox. While he examined my leg in detail, we slipped back into our usual merry banter. But this time my light mood was genuine. I really felt carefree and light-hearted, not pretending to be jolly in order to please Mr Lennox. He was just saying something flat-tering about my next twenty-five years while examining my right groin, which he had not done since our first encounter thirteen months before, when he abruptly stopped talking, leaving an incompleted sentence in mid-air. I immediately remembered Jane Zorza's case history – melanoma spreading from foot to groin – and my heart gave a violent lurch.

'I hope you haven't found anything nasty?' I asked as coolly as I could manage.

He paused before answering. 'There is a small node in your groin,' he said. 'It's quite small, probably only a swollen lymph gland. But we'll have to keep an eye on it.' Where had all my blood gone? I felt ice cold and my middle, from my lower jaw to the pit of my stomach, was trembling, gripped by sheer terror of a kind I had not felt before. And I could not get any comfort from Mr Lennox who had already moved across the room to wash his hands.

'Could this be another . . . malignancy?' I managed to ask at last.

'We can't exclude that possibility. But, as I say, it may be something utterly harmless.' He turned round to face me. 'I don't want you to probe your groin,' he said in his familiar didactic voice. 'I want you to leave it strictly alone. Don't even touch it. Let's give it a fortnight and see if it disappears. I'd like to see you as soon as Christmas is over – better make an appointment with my secretary now.' He gave me a tense smile. 'Above all don't worry and enjoy your Christmas.'

'Enjoy it?' Was this man completely inhuman or completely lacking in imagination? 'How do you expect me to enjoy my Christmas with this uncertainty hanging over me? Knowing that I may be in trouble again? Last Christmas was bad enough, but then at least I knew where I was, and now I don't!'

Mr Lennox raised his eyebrows. 'There's no need for you to get upset,' he said evenly. 'You have a great deal of discipline – why don't you use it to make yourself forget about that node until you come back to see me? Just put it out of your mind.'

Thank you, Mr Lennox. Merry Christmas, Mr

Lennox, all the very best. See you on the 29th. No, of course, there is nothing to worry about.

Numb, numb. Once again I walked along Bond Street, but this time I moved like a clockwork toy about to run down. A great numbness had settled on me like a cushion of fog, deadening all sound and movement. My body was ticking over, but only just, with shallow breathing, badly focussing eyes, a sensation of slowed down circulation, and in the middle of it all the uncontrollable trembling of sheer animal fear. I caught a glimpse of myself in a shop window and saw a white face with blank eyes. I turned off Bond Street and went to a small café for shelter. Coffee, toast, cigarette: oral comfort, dummies for the scared middle-aged baby suffering from shock and exposure. Exposure to doom. My brain, like a deranged squirrel, kept leaping around from thought to image to memory and back again. Jane Zorza's fate clashed with Mr Lennox's many assurances of my cancer-free future; my own sense of fitness and high spirits of only an hour before was now clashing with the dark fear that my body was sheltering some hostile process that would eventually destroy it.

It was a desperately lonely moment in that scruffy little café. Even its noisy, warm atmosphere, smelly with coffee and fried onions, somehow managed to flow around me without touching that desolate stillness within. Being that scared was like being trapped inside a huge ice cube. I wanted Hudie, I wanted my mother and Catherine and John and all the other people I loved to come and surround me and hold me tight and say that it would be all right, they would not let me come to any harm.

I paid and left the café.

As soon as I got to my office, I locked my door and, disregarding Mr Lennox's instructions, examined my right groin. Yes, there was a small, hard node fairly deep below the surface, roughly the shape and size of an almond. It did not hurt. If I had not looked for it, I would never have known it was there. How long had it been there? What would it do next? Launch me on the same inexorable journey to death that Jane Zorza had endured, only more slowly because I was twice her age? Above all, for God's sake, what business did it have to be there when Mr Lennox had cut so much off my right leg precisely to prevent any further doom?

Somehow I managed to re-balance myself and get through the rest of the day, without losing my composure. But after work, when I met Catherine in our usual wine bar, I poured out the bad news at once. The place was empty. We sat in the large bay window, facing the rainy darkness outside, and I could feel the tears rising from somewhere deep towards my eyes. Whatever else this cancer was doing to me, it had certainly taught me to cry after a lifetime of dry-eyed coping. All right, I thought, let it come. My first tear plopped into the house wine. Then, after a while, I finished my story.

Catherine sat silently for a moment. 'What is it you're most afraid of?' she asked at last. 'What's the worst thing that could happen to you in this situation?'

'Not death,' I said. 'You know that. Death would be like going home. But I haven't been reckoning with that possibility until now. What I'm terribly afraid of is having to go through the same torture as that poor Zorza girl before dying anyway – being chopped up and patched up and chopped some more until nothing else can be removed and they put a screen round your bed or send you home. I don't want that.'

'Of course not. And what is it you do want?'

I gulped some wine to hold down the next wave of crying. What did I want beside not having cancer, a choice that was not on the menu? 'If this node is a secondary cancer,' I said slowly, thinking aloud, 'I don't want any further surgery. I'd like to try some alternative, holistic therapy if there is a promising one. And if that doesn't work and there's no hope then I want to be taken to a hospice and seen out gently and with dignity.

83

Like Jane, but without all the pointless medical torture she had to suffer first.'

'I wish you hadn't read that wretched book.' Catherine sounded angry. 'It's given you the worst possible expectations. What happened to that poor girl needn't happen to you – no two cases are exactly alike, are they?'

'No, but even so I'm glad I read the book. I've learnt a lot from it. For instance, it made me understand why both the dermatologist and Lennox immediately examined my groin when I first called on them; melanoma tends to metastasize into the lymph glands before it spreads further. Anyway, that's my conclusion. Honestly, I'm glad I did my homework. Perhaps if I'd had a node in my groin a year ago, Lennox wouldn't have operated on my leg.'

'Or he would have chopped up your leg *and* your groin.' Catherine put her warm hand on my icy one. 'Look, if the node is harmless, there's no problem, and it bothers me that you seem to dismiss that possibility . . . it's not like you to expect the worst. But all right, supposing the node is malignant and supposing that there is no effective alternative therapy – would you consider killing yourself?'

'At present I don't think I would. I'm still haunted by that powerful dream I had some years ago – I dreamt I had killed myself and had to face my judges in the underworld, a very Egyptian kind of underworld, too . . . and the judges were furious with me because I'd tried to escape from some unfinished ghastly situation, which wasn't permissible – I still remember the shock of being stuck in limbo between life and death, unable to reach either. And those huge judges: they looked like large sandstone statues, but they spoke and moved their heads. That dream put me off suicide. But when I dreamt it I was in perfect health. I don't know what I'd say if I were terminally ill. Perhaps I'd beg to be allowed to kill myself.'

Catherine thought for a while. We emptied our glasses. The place was beginning to fill up. 'If I promise you,' Catherine said at last, 'that whatever happens and whatever you decide to do, John and I will help and support you to the limit of our ability, will you feel less frightened? If I promise you that we won't abandon you under any circumstances and will help you to stay in this world or get out of it, depending on your wishes, will you feel better?'

I nodded. There was no need for words. My despair already felt less solid, less oppressive. I held on to Catherine's hand. She was my true and unflinching ally, a comrade in arms who would no more abandon me than I would forsake her. It was a moment of experiencing unconditional, open-ended friendship, which had long been my highest value, and it comforted me deeply.

'Thank you,' I said. 'I hope I'll never have to ask you to get me poison or razor blades or whatever one needs. I'd rather sit it out, whatever it's going to be. But I'm grateful to have the option to go, with your help. Hudie would never help me to do away with myself, I know that. He'd do just about anything for me, he'd move mountains, but he'd never help me to commit suicide.'

'A lot of people would agree with him about that.'

'I know, I know. Hudie hasn't come to terms with death, not even in general, let alone with mine. Will you promise to stand by him if I die? We're so very close and he's invested all his feelings into our relationship. He'd take it very badly if I went.'

'Well then, you'd better not die. Save us all a lot of trouble. But of course we'll stand by him. Whether he'll accept help is a different matter. Are you going to tell him about all this?'

'Not for the time being. I've already told him on the 'phone today that Lennox had found everything in good order. If the node is cancerous, we might just as well have a last undisturbed Christmas together. If it's harmless, he need never know about this panic. In fact, you're the only one who knows about it.'

Already I was thinking in pairs of alternatives. If I live, if I die – a constant weighing of polarities that soon became an automatic habit. Oddly enough, it reassured me: thinking along parallel lines brought order to my inner chaos. If I live, if I die; it was like the even balance required for skating, one foot life, one foot death, glide along on both with total equanimity, without bias. I did not even consider the third possibility of long, lingering invalidism. What I knew about melanoma made anything long-term seem unlikely.

When the barman put on his noisiest tape, we wandered off and had a vaguely Italian meal in a considerably brighter mood. Eventually we parted in Gloucester Road like on so many previous occasions, like on the evening, over a year ago, when the threat of cancer had first nudged me. In the train I contemplated what I saw as Catherine's samurai streak: a clear, steely quality of absolute courage and calm that somehow co-existed with her womanly warmth and caring. It seemed a strange mixture, but only at a first glance and only in the mode of either-or thinking. In terms of and-and, which was the way we were both trying to live, aiming for wholeness and roundedness, Catherine was simply more integrated than anybody else I knew, standing at the mid-point of her polarities and letting them seesaw. But now, after that harrowing day, I meditated on that quality of Catherine's that linked her with the ancient swordmasters of Japan – a compound of wisdom, skill, unflinching courage and grace. Just to tune into that helped to uncrumple my spine and keep it straight, at least until my next confrontation with Mr Lennox. And that was seventeen days away.

The only way I was able to handle the intervening period was in the 'As if . . .' mode, acting as if all were well, normal, perfectly fine. The trick worked. My poise only faltered when some unsuspecting friend or colleague joyfully told me how much better off I was than I had been a year before – no more hospital Christmas pudding, no more pain. But those brief tremors passed quickly. What did not pass was the node in my groin which I gingerly checked every day. If anything, it felt slightly bigger. But I had no other symptoms.

On my last working day before the Christmas break I was just about to lock up my office when the plastic identity card, worn on a chain round my neck, broke and fell on the floor for no obvious reason. Of course plastic can, and often does, spontaneously crack, I knew that. But my basic instinctual self, the one that notices strange coincidences and picks up telepathic information without really trying, responded with a superstitious shudder. Did the broken disc forecast the end of my professional identity? Was I on the way out from my scruffy, much-loved office with its windowsill jungle and highly personal decorations? I mended the plastic disc with a piece of sticky tape and put it back round my neck. Then I took it off again and went home.

Christmas with Hudie was outwardly beautiful. Inside my tension was growing day by day. I needed more and more energy to hold down the lid and not shout my fears at the top of my voice. On the 27th, which was a mild, anticlimatic Saturday, I finally ran out of energy and self-control and I desperately wanted Hudie to go back to his flat so that I could take off my mask, have a good howl, get drunk or go to sleep. I began to pace up and down, up and down, choking, wondering how to break the deadlock without breaking anything else.

'All right, darling,' Hudie said quietly. 'Why don't you sit down and tell me about it?'

I did. I do not remember how we spent the rest of that weekend, except that we sat for a long time huddled together in silence, watching the early dusk take over the room.

On Sunday night, barely twelve hours before going to see Mr Lennox, I dreamt about him. In the dream we met in a weird, deserted town where most of the buildings were damaged or in ruins. 'Let me give you dinner,' he said. 'I'm a good cook. I always do the cooking when my wife is away.' He beckoned me to his stately, distinctly pre-war car and, to my dismay, made me take the back seat from where I could only see his back. After a short drive we got out at a roofless house that had only three walls and was full of rubble. An ancient kitchen range stood in the middle of all that desolation, and Mr Lennox began to cook dinner on it. He went through a number of complicated operations at great speed, performing them with the aplomb of a stage magician – mixing, chopping, blending, stirring and sousing. I watched him with fascination, feeling more and more ravenous. At last he handed me a large dinner plate, with a tiny, off-putting smudge of unidentifiable food on it. I looked at the plate, feeling bitterly disappointed. Is this all? I thought; after all those preparations and displays of skill, is this all the nourishment he is offering me? I decided not to touch that nasty small mess. And I woke up.

I promptly replayed the dream behind my closed eyelids. Well, well, so that is what I really felt about Mr Lennox's skills and services – my unconscious seemed to have reached a decision about my medical problem well before the conscious brain, and even before I officially knew that I had a problem. And, as always, I had to bow to the unconscious for the artistry and accuracy of its symbolic language: the ruined city and the obsolete car and kitchen range it had assigned to Mr Lennox added up to a comment that my conscious mind found disturbingly sharp. So I recorded the dream but put it out of my mind for the time being.

Long before Christmas Catherine had offered to accompany me to Mr Lennox and I had accepted. ('Women handle these situations better,' I had told

Hudie, who had wanted to go with me, too.) Now, after my powerful dream, I was doubly glad to have Catherine with me to act as an objective, perceptive witness and stop me from getting things out of proportion. Part of me, I realised, already saw Mr Lennox as a thin, quiet angel of death or at least as a harbinger of great trouble, and I did not want to slide into even worse distortion.

Catherine and I met on Mr Lennox's doorstep, hugged, and then sat in the waiting-room, barely speaking. I knew she had cancelled her day's workload to be with me, but in my frozen terror I did not feel guilty, only deeply grateful to have her there, my secret samurai disguised as an elegant woman in a Rodier two-piece.

Half past twelve. Up those gently curving period stairs once more. Introductions. No, of course Mr Lennox did not mind my friend's presence, on the contrary. We sat briefly in his study, he consulted his notes and then led me next door, to the examination couch. My stomach felt like a ton of cold lead. I did not have to wait long. He probed my groin, withdrew his hand and said, 'Yes, it's still there. Would you like to get dressed? Let's go next door and discuss the next step.'

Damn you, I thought, that is one way to tell me the worst – not the way I would have chosen personally. We returned to his consulting room and sat down. That dreadful uncontrollable shaking was creeping up my middle again, making my lower jaw unsteady. Mr Lennox contemplated his interlaced fingers and then looked at me.

'We must establish what that node is,' he said. 'That means a biopsy involving the removal of the lymph gland. If the node is malignant, I'll arrange for a whole body scan to see whether there are any other metastases. If we don't find anything else, which I hope will be the case, I'll remove all the lymph glands from the right groin area.'

'Good God,' I exclaimed, remembering the intense pain in my still swollen right foot where only a few lymph glands were missing. 'If you remove all the glands, how will the lymph circulate?'

'It won't, I'm afraid. Your right leg will be permanently swollen and you'll have to wear support tights for the rest of your life.'

I felt anger rising to my throat. What is the matter with this man? I wondered: first he cuts off part of my leg, then he makes it swell up for life. What kind of a cure is that, especially if the second operation turns out to be as useless as . . . ? I did not allow myself to complete the question. The enormity of the situation squashed my anger. What I wanted to know was why Lennox was looking at me so grimly, almost accusingly, as if I had committed a crime or at least a heinous sin by developing a lump in my groin. Should I not shout and swear at him for having lulled me into false security before tipping me out of it, onto a bed of scalpels and pain?

'I know you have private health insurance,' Mr Lennox went on, 'but I'd like you to come to the general ward of the National Health Service hospital where I work, not to the private hospital where you went last year.'

I looked at him in amazement. Catherine said quietly, 'My friend has a very great need for privacy, especially under stress. I don't think she'd last long in a public ward.'

'Oh yes, I'm sure she would. And I could give her better care.'

'I thought you gave me excellent care in my private room,' I said. 'Frankly, I see no earthly reason why I should go to your general ward when I have the option of a single room. But don't let's go into details. I want to find my bearings first. All this is very difficult and

90

totally unexpected. After all, you've been telling me for the past year that I was fine, and now this. What I want to know is . . . if you operate and remove my lymph glands . . .' I had to stop and take a deep breath to steady my voice. 'If you operate, what are my chances of not developing another tumour elsewhere?'

He hesitated. 'I'd say about sixty per cent,' he said at last. And I knew that he was not telling the truth.

'That's not much better than fifty-fifty. Not very impressive, is it? And what happens if you don't operate and we do nothing?'

'I'd give you between six weeks and six months.' Now at last I had received payment in full for having insisted on knowing the truth right from the start. It was a brutal kind of payment, too, but then Mr Lennox's whole manner seemed to have changed, and even his face appeared unfamiliar. His eyes looked dull and cold, he had withdrawn into an area of personal permafrost. He did not have a word or gesture of comfort or encouragement for me, only that accusing look which suggested that I had let the side down and deserved what was coming to me. We all rose, as if a trumpet had blasted the meeting to an end. Catherine took hold of my hand.

'Is there no alternative to surgery?' she asked. 'No other treatment?'

'I'm afraid there isn't. Neither radiotherapy nor chemotherapy works in cases such as this. Surgery holds out the best hope.'

Some hope, I thought. Is it any better than the hope you gave me before, and anyway, for God's sake, what is this all about? But I was unable to speak.

'I want to do the biopsy within a week,' Mr Lennox said. 'Will you make an appointment now?'

'No, not now. I'll ring your secretary later.'

He let us go. Down in the street, in the very heart of that well-groomed medical quarter, I felt a rush of poignant sympathy for the thousands before me who had walked along that same street in a state of shock similar to mine, crushed by the weight of a grim diagnosis and no hope. *Ave Caesar, morituri te saluant.*

We went to my favourite café in Wigmore Street. It was crowded – we had to share a table with two inane, giggling girls – so we ate fast and talked very little. Every now and then a sob rose from my chest but passed unnoticed in the general hubbub. After the meal Catherine hailed a cab and we drove to her flat on the edge of Primrose Hill.

The bare trees on the top of the hill rose from a veil of thin mist with the starkness of a Japanese pen drawing. The sight absorbed and almost hypnotised me. First from the road and then from Catherine's window I had to look at it, sink into it, become part of it, to the exclusion of all else. Perhaps those thin dark lines separated by thick white spaces provided the perfect pattern to act as a visual shock absorber and brief refuge. Trees again, I thought, trees as saviours, just like those plane trees seen from the hospital window last year. And then even the thoughts stopped and only the looking remained.

Catherine tucked me up in a nest of cushions on her sofa. She put a warm rug around me and handed me a cup of lemon tea richly laced with brandy. She waited until I had finished my contemplation of the trees and drunk my tea and then said, 'Your colour is normal again. How do you feel? Would you like to rest for a while or do you feel like talking?'

'I don't want to rest, thanks.'

'All right then, let's talk. What are you going to do?'

'I don't know. Run away. No, that's not true. I'd like the whole business to unhappen so that we could relax and talk about something else. Oh, sorry, I'm talking nonsense. What am I going to do? Not have further surgery, I think. It seems pointless.'

'While you were being examined, I took a quick look at Lennox's notes. Apparently everything was fine until

92

your last check-up. I think he was nearly as shocked as you when he found that the node was still there.'

'Shocked? Do you really think he was shocked? All I could pick up was terrible coldness and disapproval, as if I'd committed something unforgivable instead of being the victim. One of the reasons why I went to pieces was precisely the feeling of being completely rejected by him . . . we used to talk about all manner of things, about his son's doings and my various preoccupations and hobbies, and even on Christmas Day he visited me in the hospital . . . and now, when I most needed support, he didn't show me a scrap of humanity.'

'Because that's the only way he can deal with a painful situation,' Catherine said. 'You must have noticed how completely out of touch he is with his feelings; no doubt if he were in touch with them, he couldn't function as a surgeon. Or, to go even further back, why did he become a surgeon and not a physician? However, I'm not really concerned with Mr Lennox's psyche. One day you'll have to work through your feelings towards him, but not now. So you don't want more surgery?'

'The way I feel now, no, I don't, unless it's absolutely necessary.'

'Then you'll have to try alternative medicine. Do you have anything in mind?'

'No, nothing specific. None of the alternative therapies I'm familiar with has a coherent anti-cancer programme. And melanoma spreads so fast that there's no time to experiment.'

Catherine picked up her large address book. 'Before you make any decision, you need a second opinion and possibly a third one, from physicians, not surgeons, who are open-minded. We must also find out about alternative cancer therapies and look at them. Why don't you relax while I make a few 'phone calls?'

It was like being a child again, a well-nursed sick

child enjoying perfect comfort and care. Warmth, early dusk, soft cushions, hot drinks, and the presence of my friend added up to a sense of security. I was aware of Catherine's voice in the background and of the sound of repeated dialling, but I let my mind drift without listening. I only emerged from my reverie when she sat down next to me and handed me a list of names and telephone numbers.

'We're doing well,' she said. 'Here are the names of two physicians who are sympathetic to alternative methods. You should go and see them as soon as possible. Then I spoke to Ann Procter – remember her? You did the counselling training together. Ann has many talents. She is a qualified social worker, a teacher of relaxation and a healer and also a glider pilot, although the latter isn't of immediate relevance to us. But Ann also knows a great deal about holistic medicine, and she thinks you should take a look at the Gerson therapy.'

'Oh? Did she say what that's about?'

'Only that it's nutritionally based. And that you should contact somebody called Margaret Straus who can brief you about the therapy. She's the London contact. I gather that the Gerson centre itself is in the United States. All the names and numbers are on the list. Will this do for a start?'

'Oh yes, thank you!' I gazed at the list. 'Years ago,' I told Catherine, 'when fate versus free will was a constant topic among my friends, I evolved my Clapham Junction theory. It went like this: at moments of crisis we are faced with a number of alternatives that are like tracks at a vast railway junction, all bunched together and equally available. So we choose one, and that's free will. But then that's it, we've got to follow it right through, each track ending up elsewhere. And that's fate. It's a pretty weak theory, simply asking to be shot down on various grounds, but even so I feel I've reached a typical Clapham Junction moment, and I'm not ready to choose.'

'Which tracks are you considering at present?'

'Track One: Lennox, surgery, a messy end . . . why should a second operation do the trick when the first one didn't, and when the cancer has had a whole year to spread and strike roots? Track Two: refuse treatment, sort out my affairs, resign my job, travel and do all the things I've been longing to do.'

'That alone might cure you, you know. Track Three?'

'Going alternative. Try Gerson or whatever, and take the consequences.'

'At least that's a manageable choice. So, what are you going to do about it?'

I had to laugh. What-are-you-going-to-do-about-it was one of Catherine's great phrases, always spoken firmly yet gently over the years in reply to one of my periodic dirges concerning some intractable problem. At first, years before, I had fallen for the deceptive lightness of her voice and had explained, with some passion, why I was unable to do anything about it. But back it had come, the same question in the same clear and caring voice, this time asking me what I was going to do about my inability to act. Becoming able to act or else accepting the problem without further yowling were two possibilities implied, though never put into words.

'What am I going to do about it? I'm going to ask you to make appointments for me with those two doctors. Without seeing them I can't decide on anything. And just now I can't talk coherently to strangers.'

Both doctors agreed to see me on New Year's Eve, a timing I found interesting – last chance consultations on the last day of a year that had started with sickness and pain, and was ending in confusion. Then I rang Hudie and asked him to meet us in a nearby pub. Catherine and I walked there through the dark streets, both of us emotionally exhausted. Yet we still had to break the news to Hudie, explain and cushion the shock. It was a heavy, painful hour, only slightly eased by brandy and sharing. Then Catherine went home while we walked through St John's Wood in search of a snack. As we passed a bare street tree, a blackbird began to sing directly overhead and went on for several minutes in the late December night when, as far as I know, blackbirds are not supposed to pour out their best music. But that bird did not know the rules and it trilled, piped and throbbed in an ecstasy of sound. We stood and listened, enthralled. That birdsong was as unseasonal as the solitary golden daisy had been over a year ago. It did not solve any problems. But it provided some consolation.

5

THE NEXT MORNING, feeling somewhat calmer, I rang Margaret Straus, the London contact for information on the Gerson therapy. I expected a stately, elderly voice to answer but heard a young and pleasant American one instead, and discovered that Ms Straus was the grand-daughter of Dr Gerson who had himself died in New York in 1959. I told her about my problem. She agreed to see me, but only after I had read, or at least skimmed through, two American books which contained all the necessary information on the therapy. Once I had understood the basic principles, she would be glad to answer my questions.

In my shocked and restless state I would have preferred to consult her at once. But I saw her point and dashed out to get the two books. Once was *A Cancer Therapy – Results of Fifty Cases* by Max Gerson, MD, a hefty volume in a bright royal blue cover. The grim photographs and ghostly X-ray pictures illustrating the case histories made me a little uncomfortable – I felt I was trespassing on medical territory where I had no business to be. The main text looked rather technical, so I started on the other, much thinner book which promised to be an easier read. *Cancer Victor – How I Purged Myself of Melanoma* was by Jaquie Davison, and while the Gerson book had intimidated me with its gravity, this one seemed far too lightweight, written in the breathless style of well-meaning but naive health magazines. However, if the author had really healed herself of what she kept calling deadly melanoma – it

bothered me to see my disease described so starkly –
then I had to find out how she had done it.

There was not much going on at work, so I was able
to do some fast, concentrated reading. At first, Jaquie
Davison came across as a nice, naive, gushing woman,
a Christian fundamentalist with an intense, childish
relationship to her God. Moreover, she was a fervent
believer in the traditional role of women and a leading
opponent of the Equal Rights Amendment in the United
States. That last fact alone was enough to put my back
up, but I read on, and gradually my respect for the
woman's courage cancelled out my irritation. She had
been overwhelmed by melanoma at the age of thirty-
six, with tumours proliferating all over her body (the
largest one sitting in her right groin – oh Lord, that
right groin again). It had been too late for any conventional treatment. Besides, the ghastly cancer deaths of
some of her relatives had put Mrs Davison off orthodox
medicine. And so, after some trials and errors, after
preparing to die within two months, she decided to try
the Gerson therapy at home, with the help of her
devoted husband and fourteen-year-old daughter who
took a year off from school to attend her mother.

The therapy, I discovered from the book, consisted of
a strict vegetarian diet with huge amounts of freshly
made raw vegetable and fruit juices, and drastic detoxification by means of frequent coffee enemas. Coffee
enemas? Any enema was vile, I remembered that from
my early childhood, but coffee enemas sounded particularly revolting. Why coffee? And why take them so
frequently? I had many other questions but from
Jaquie's highly subjective, rhapsodic account it was
hard to discern the therapeutic principles behind the
strange details. But her progress was so dramatic,
spiced with several near-fatal crises, that I felt it best to
suspend my disbelief and even my critical faculty in
order to read to the end before starting to ask questions.

Jaquie's story, told so artlessly, was remarkable. She

had persevered for two years against deadly odds, against all reason and medical expectations, without skilled help, trusting in God and in the late Dr Gerson's ideas, and she had won. Clearly, her totally committed fundamentalist approach had given her the strength to persevere. Equally clearly, that approach had advantages over my own critical, sceptical, 'yes-but' attitude. Now, too, despite my admiration for a very brave woman I experienced a surge of scepticism, a vague disappointment with the therapy itself. Raw vegetable juices and enemas against cancer sounded like slings and arrows against a nuclear warhead. Yes, I knew that naturopaths, using diet alone, were successfully treating chronic diseases and I knew people whose severe arthritis, migraine, high blood pressure or diabetes had dramatically improved on nature cure diets. But surely cancer was in a class of its own and had to be fought with something more potent than the gallons of carrot and apple juice that Jaquie Davison seemed to have drunk day and night for such a long time?

Ah yes, but Jaquie had recovered. By the time I finished her book in the evening, I felt a kind of friendship for her, and some faint hope for myself, for my disease seemed much less advanced than hers had been at the outset, and so, perhaps, if I decided to follow the Gerson therapy . . .

All right. Better find out more about it.

I poured myself a drink, lit a cigarette and opened Dr Gerson's book at random. 'Forbidden,' it said in heavy capitals, 'Nicotine, salt, alcohol,' followed by a long list of banned foods, including meat, eggs, fish, cheese, butter, milk, all processed foods, all fats and oils, tea, coffee, chocolate, cream, nuts, mushrooms, spices, and even ordinary drinking water. But, above all, nicotine, salt, alcohol. Never mind the salt, I thought, swirling around the whisky in my glass and gazing at the blue smoke of my filter-tipped, low tar, utterly sensible cigarette. Never mind the salt or even the frozen spinach, it is one or two other things that would be very, very tough to give up. But I started to read and was hooked by the first sentence of the introduction: 'This book has been written to indicate that there is an effective treatment of cancer, even in advanced cases.'

Two hours later I had to stop reading. My eyes were no longer focussing and I was experiencing the shock of a totally new insight that was astounding in its simplicity; an insight that, if it was correct, would compel me to revise all my ideas about health and sickness. I needed time and space to digest all that new information. Reading the book had been like listening to a voice, a precise, scholarly and modest voice explaining the thinking behind a lifetime's work. But that same modest voice also made some staggering claims, and the case histories, filling the second half of the book, apparently substantiated them. They seemed to prove that the German-born Dr Gerson, working on his own, had really found an effective cancer treatment, and had written a book to tell the world how to do it. I was feeling deeply stirred, not quite believing what I was reading.

At that moment Catherine rang, wanting to know how I was and what life felt like after the previous day's upheavals.

'I'm fine, just a little tired,' I said. 'But I can't go to bed because I've got to read Dr Gerson's book as fast as I can. Margaret Straus won't see me until I've read it. And it's rather long.'

'But is it interesting?'

'Mind-blowing,' I said. 'Totally original. If Dr Gerson is right, then there's something wrong with a lot of current cancer treatments. Mind you, I only started reading two hours ago, but I think I've got the main drift of his reasoning. And it's beautifully logical.'

'Oh good,' said Catherine. 'I'm glad you sound so

enthusiastic. Are you thinking of trying the therapy yourself?'

'I don't know yet. First I've got to finish the book and meet Margaret Straus. I mustn't get carried away. But if Gerson's claims are true, then his therapy should be standard treatment everywhere.'

Catherine chuckled. 'Oh, come,' she said. 'If his treatment works and if it's as original as you say, then surely the Establishment will do its best to suppress it – isn't that the classic reaction? Still, never mind the Establishment, as long as you think that the therapy might help you.'

'Well, I'll discuss that tomorrow with the two doctors you've rounded up for me. You see, I want to make up my mind one way or the other before the year is out.'

'Well, that leaves you exactly twenty-six hours. I'd better let you get on with that book. But please ring me any time you feel like talking.'

I returned to my vigil.

Time was short. I had to concentrate on understanding Dr Gerson's basic ideas as they emerged from the rich and complex material of his book, so I began to jot them down, just as if I had been doing some last-minute research for an urgent, overdue script. My notes went like this:

'Cancer is not a specific localised disease but a general, chronic, degenerative one. Therefore it is useless to remove tumours or try to eradicate other symptoms. They will only recur in a different location.

'Moreover, cancer is not so much a disease as a symptom, the symptom of a sick body with a damaged metabolism and a broken-down immune system. The correct treatment is to restore the body to normal healthy functioning so that it can destroy and discard the cancer by itself. Healthy bodies are able to prevent their cells from turning abnormal, i.e. malignant.

'Metabolism and immune system are gradually damaged over a long period of time by inadequate nutrition:

101

food grown in a depleted, artificially fertilised soil that does not contain the necessary minerals; food deficient in proteins and potassium, made toxic by chemicals, processed and refined until it contains no live, active nutrients without which health cannot be maintained. The malnourished body is then made even more toxic by environmental pollution: impure air and water, chemicals at large everywhere. Eventually the hidden starvation and the accumulation of toxins combine to cause a breakdown in the body's defence system, so that a tumour can develop.

'The degenerative process leading to cancer involves most of the vital organs. You cannot get cancer unless your liver, pancreas, kidneys and bile system are impaired. All bodily processes work together and are deranged together in disease. Thus, all processes have to be brought back to normal and healed.

'In order to heal the body, it must be detoxified and activated with ionised minerals and natural, organically grown food, so that the vital organs can function again.'

I read my notes and then closed my eyes to rest them. The book's simple message was sending powerful shockwaves through my mind. Besides, I was intrigued and slightly appalled by some of the information I had just soaked up: for instance, that cancer cells were throwbacks, revenants from an ancient phase of evolution, obeying sinister laws that did not apply to normal cells. For one thing, cancer cells multiplied as fast as the cells of an embryo which develops at vast speed from a fertilised ovum. But while the embryonic cells knew when to slow down, cancer cells did not and so eventually destroyed their host. For another thing those greedy, disorganised cells thrived on fermentation, like all life forms must have done in an unimaginably remote, primitive stage of evolution, before the Earth acquired its present atmosphere. My mind's eye promptly visualised a bleak planetscape, a kind of pre-Earth consisting of desolate, dun-coloured mud; and the only signs of life on that airless lump were evil bubbles rising from the fermenting primeval slime. Fermentation versus oxidation, rotting versus breathing, primitive, uncontrolled rogue cells rising from the depths to overrun our sophisticated evolved bodies – the process formed a gruesome parallel to the psychological disaster which occurs when dark, unconscious contents overwhelm and destroy our daytime consciousness and rational mind. Was it sheer chance that schizophrenics rarely contracted cancer? Did one breakdown exclude the other? There was something deeply disquieting in this doubly emphasised regressive nature of cancer cells. Since the development of the embryo repeated the evolutionary phases of the human race, condensing millions of years into nine months, the earliest, fastest rate of cell division corresponded to our most remote biological past, just as the fermenting mud belonged to the most remote past of our planet. How weird and ironical that cancer should grow into an intractable epidemic in our part of the world at the precise moment when Western technology is soaring from peak to peak and our early beginnings seem remote enough to be denied. It was as if Nature was sending a message through the cells of our bodies to say that something was wrong, that our cells were regressing into morbid chaos because we were allowing our soaring technology to interfere with our food and lifestyle in a way that our bodies could not tolerate.

It was nearly midnight. My house was so quiet that it might have been a houseboat anchored in some deserted dream lake, and I sat stock still within that great silence, trying to reach some conclusion. I felt I was standing on a razor-sharp boundary between two mutually exclusive alternatives, carrying my disease both on my back and inside my body; and I knew that I would have to step off that dangerous borderline before it cut off my feet.

If Dr Gerson is right, I thought, and I suspect he is, if

it really is useless to remove tumours unless they are life-threatening, then my operation was useless, all that pain and suffering and mutilation were totally futile, further surgery would be equally senseless, and Mr Lennox does not know what the hell he is doing. Or perhaps he does, perhaps he realises that his virtuoso skills can bring no cure but he carries on all the same because he does not know what else to do. And if that is so, may God forgive him, because I can not.

If cancer is really a disease of the entire metabolism, then the only way to tackle it is to heal and restore that metabolism. If Dr Gerson is right, then there is no other way to survive.

The more I pondered the therapy, the more sense it made. Everything I had ever heard and seen of conventional orthodox cancer treatment flashed through my mind like a jumbled up film run at twice the normal speed. Friends, acquaintances and neighbours trailing from operation to treatment and back again, looking like bloodless, egg-bald survivors of some death camp after courses of chemotherapy; growing skeletal, smelling of death long before dying, dying at last long after hope had died. I caught a memory flash of my beautiful little schoolmate, Alexandra, who died of cancer of the mouth at the age of ten, and how we all went to her funeral and how I felt ill for days afterwards, unable to get rid of the heavy, sickly smell that had overpowered the scent of the flowers covering her coffin. I thought of Jane Zorza and her sad, helpless dying. All those victims had received orthodox treatment. I did not know of anyone who had attempted some unorthodox method, except for Dr Gerson's fifty cases. Perhaps I should attempt it myself.

Only thirty-six hours had passed since my last meeting with Mr Lennox, but it felt like a week. I decided not to decide anything and went to sleep.

The next morning I told my bosses what was happening and asked for time off for medical appointments. It was a painful conversation. My feelings were so exposed that their kindness and sympathy plunged me into tearfulness. I also realised that what I had told them was doom-laden by definition and that they thought I was going to die. At any rate, they gave me *carte blanche* in matters of appointments and even offered to take me off my current anthropological programme which I refused, and then we all went to the canteen for a coffee and a sticky bun because we could not think of anything else.

After lunch I left the office and went to see Dr Montague, the first of the two reputedly open-minded physicians recommended by Catherine's contacts. It is a bit of a gamble, I thought, trekking towards his house under a pall of weariness. How open is open-minded, how do I discover where the boundaries are? But when I reached the quiet waiting-room, my apprehension lifted. The room had a sheltering air, the fascinating books on the shelves betrayed a wide range of non-medical interests, and in a corner there was a battered, sad-unto-death teddy bear, slouched against a splendid cushion. Oh God, I know how you feel, I said to it inwardly, wondering where my own childhood teddy, the plump and glossy Shoomie, might be – if indeed he was still anywhere. I also fought off a powerful urge to pick up that despondent creature and give it a hug. But beneath that brief diversion I was very frightened.

Dr Montague turned out to be soft-spoken, courteous and very serious, to the point of appearing almost sad. He was slightly built with fine bones, of indeterminate age, possessing a quality of gentleness that came across obliquely, filtered by his reserve. He took my complete medical history, carried out a general examination and finally concentrated on the enlarged gland in my groin. 'Yes, I feel certain that this is a cancerous growth,' he said at last. 'There's little point in having a biopsy which often causes the cancer to spread.' He looked at my mutilated right leg with its large, permanently dark red

105

skin graft which, after more than a year, still looked like a dreadful, angry wound. 'After that experience you have every right to oppose further surgery,' he said, so quietly that I had to strain to hear him. 'What do you intend to do about your illness?'

Heavens, I thought, how marvellous to be asked instead of receiving orders. I said, 'I'm thinking of trying the Gerson therapy because it sounds eminently logical and rational. Do you happen to know about it?'

I was in luck. Dr Montague swivelled round towards the bookshelf behind his desk and pulled out the familiar royal blue volume. 'Yes, I've read Gerson's book and found it most interesting, but I've had no practical experience with his therapy. I must say it sounds a very tough regime.'

'Frankly, I haven't reached the practical details yet, but I find his thinking fascinating. It makes sense. I'll know more about the practice when I've met his grand-daughter who lives in London. I may see her in a day or two.' I paused for a moment. 'Perhaps it's too early to ask you, but . . . if I decide to go on the therapy, would you be willing to provide medical supervision?'

He hesitated. 'Well . . . yes, as long as it's understood that I've had no practical experience with this therapy.'

'Of course. I don't expect many doctors have. Look, I've no great expectations, I know that choosing this therapy is a leap in the dark, but is there a good orthodox alternative that tackles the cause rather than the symptoms? No? That's what I thought. In that case I might just as well try Gerson. I intend to make up my mind by midnight about one or two things – not necessarily about all my problems – so that I don't carry too much muddle over into the New Year.'

Dr Montague listened gravely, not trying to advise or influence me in any way, and from the quality of his listening I knew that he would grant me space and freedom to make my own decision in peace. I also accepted with a sense of finality that there really was no orthodox solution to my problem, and that going the unorthodox way might be only marginally less lonely than dying.

'When did you last have blood and urine tests made?' Dr Montague asked.

'Oh, nearly twenty years ago, when I suffered from a hyperactive thyroid.'

'Not since? Do you mean to say that no tests have been made since the onset of the melanoma?'

When I shook my head he said nothing, but I could see that he was dismayed. I thought of Mr Lennox's total absorption in his skin graft and his total indifference to the rest of me. 'Perhaps surgeons don't believe in blood and urine tests,' I said feebly.

'I'd like you to have them done at once.' He arranged for the tests over the telephone and told me where the laboratory was; he would see me again once the results were to hand.

As I walked out into the smoky winter afternoon I felt reassured, although the doctor had not said or done anything particularly reassuring. On the contrary, he had taken away the last hope that the lump in my groin might be benign and he had offered no new, promising orthodox treatment. But despite his great reserve he had allowed me to make real contact with him, and I also sensed that he saw his patients as creatures of body, spirit and mind, not as defective organs attached to some shadowy un-person, and that in itself was reassuring.

I just made it in time to Dr Andrews, the second physician to be consulted that afternoon. He was ebullient, informal and so boyish that when he showed me in I thought he must be the doctor's son. The first thing I noticed on his desk was a mighty volume called *The Metabolic Management of Cancer*. For the second time that afternoon I recited my full medical history, underwent a full examination, and was told that a biopsy was superfluous; the node in my groin was undoubtedly a secondary tumour and any further surgery would only make things worse.

Dr Andrews, who practised both allopathic and homoeopathic medicine, was strongly in favour of the Gerson therapy. He thought it had the best chance of success of all the alternative approaches. And it would help if I could combine it with meditation, to provide total relaxation and freedom from stress.

'No reason why I shouldn't,' I said. 'The curious thing is, I used to be a regular meditator, but some three weeks ago when I most needed tranquillity and recollection, I stopped altogether; without really noticing, almost. I suppose I channelled all my energy into staying sane and trying to make sense of my situation. As my teacher used to say, yoga comes and goes . . . so does meditation, and with me it just went.'

'You can start again now, can't you? You'll need all your inner strength if you go on the Gerson therapy. It's a long haul and very tough.'

Just before I left, Dr Andrews took a colour photograph of me and another one of my wretched right leg. 'For the record,' he said. 'You see, if you go on the therapy, after a while you'll look so much better and your leg will improve so strikingly that no one will believe how different you were if you don't have a "before" picture.'

That seemed a bit too optimistic. But I thanked him and took my leave.

Well, I thought, travelling home through the residential deserts of West London, they could not be more different, Dr Montague and Dr Andrews. One is middle-aged, reserved, intuitive, gentle and, I suspect, ultimately pessimistic; the other is young, hearty, a trifle brash and strongly optimistic. Dr Montague has the picture of a beautifully tranquil Buddha opposite his desk, Dr Andrews keeps the colour photograph of a questionable present-day guru above his mantlepiece, as if being open-minded about alternative medicine

108

went hand in hand with some interest in Oriental philosophy. They could not be more different, yet both have reached the same conclusion about my condition and outlook, and that will have to do for the time being.

Hudie came over later that evening. We had a light meal and some wine, spending a muted New Year's Eve with nothing much to celebrate. Except that as I finished telling him about my meetings with the two doctors, my heart suddenly grew lighter, my mind clearer, and without further doubts or soul-searchings I sailed into a final decision as smoothly and simply as a boat glides into harbour. It was eleven-fifteen.

'Excuse me for a few moments,' I said to Hudie. 'I must write down something while I'm in the mood.'

I went to my bedroom and wrote a note to Mr Lennox. 'After ripe reflection,' I wrote, 'I have decided to try and solve my health problem by non-surgical means. I don't expect you'll approve, but perhaps you'll wish me luck. Thank you for all your past care.'

I signed the note and took it to Hudie. 'Will you read this and tell me if it sounds too brusque or whatever?' He gazed at it and shook his head.

'No, it doesn't. If Mr Lennox takes exception to it, then he has a problem. Are you quite sure you don't want to see him again?'

'Yes, I am. There's no point in seeing him.'

'All right, then that's that. I'll support you in whatever you want to do. But please choose the right therapy so that you get well again.'

We drank to that. I had made at least one decision before 1980 was out.

I delivered my note to Mr Lennox early on the 2nd January, on my way, hungry and bleary-eyed, to undergo my tests at the medical laboratory. He was unlikely to be around so early in the morning, even more unlikely to lurk behind his front door, yet I pushed my note through the letter slot gingerly, like a child feeding a snack to a potentially dangerous dog, and almost ran down the road.

My rational mind knew that Mr Lennox was no more frightening in his person now than he had ever been, but on a less rational plane he had acquired the awful shadow of The Surgeon, the cutting, chopping, amputating archetypal bogeyman; and therefore he had to be avoided before he could inflict further wounds on me.

I did not expect to hear from him ever again, but the following day I received a reply to my note. It was twice as long as mine had been and very friendly, and as I read it, I found one sentence that really hit me between the eyes. He had written, 'I accept, only too readily, that the surgeon does not have a monopoly on the treatment of your particular problem and thus I have no right to demand, or even expect, you to follow my advice.'

Eh? What? I stomped around the house, half-astounded, half-enraged. Who was he fooling? Our last exchange in his consulting room, only five days earlier, rang loud and clear in my head, and now this –

I rang Catherine and read her the letter over the telephone, right to its kindly conclusion, 'I wish you well in your treatment and would wish to know how you progress.'

'Well, well,' said Catherine. 'Perhaps he's glad to wash his hands of you. Even so, it's a pleasant note.'

'But what about the middle bit? You remember what he told you; no other therapy was effective in a case such as mine, only surgery and nothing but surgery. And now, all of a sudden, the surgeon has no monopoly and offers blessings on my non-surgical initiative. What's this doublespeak?'

'I suppose when we saw him he spoke in his professional capacity, but when he answered your note, he wrote as a private person and therefore was able to admit that he didn't have the answer.'

'That's a charitable explanation. But I can't see it like

110

that. What I see is plain duplicity and I find it deeply upsetting, because I could have sworn that Lennox was utterly sincere and honest.'

'I'm sure he is, but his criteria are probably much more complicated than yours. The man works in a desperately sensitive area. Which patient can take how much of the truth, when is the right moment to speak – it must be a constant balancing act. Of course I can see why you're so angry. If I were in your shoes, I'd be a damn sight less understanding myself,' Catherine said.

'Does he think I'm an idiot?' I could not get over Lennox's two diametrically opposed statements. 'He said one thing in front of you, and he must have realised that you'd be a reliable witness, and now he states the exact opposite in writing, without even trying to justify such a dizzying contradiction.'

'He couldn't possibly justify it without damaging his own authority. Or even the mystique of the surgical approach. You can't expect him to do that.'

'I'd expect him to be honest at any cost. That's how we started when I first met him. Anyway, how much does his authority weigh against my survival? Oh, all right, it doesn't matter. But there's something else that's much more alarming. If I weren't capable of making my own decisions, if I were a respectful little woman – or man – who thinks that a surgeon is the nearest thing to God, I'd go along with what he suggests, undergo the biopsy, have my lymph glands ripped out and then die respectfully, without realising that my surgeon isn't even convinced that he's doing the right thing! Now that thought really frightens me.'

'Me, too. I daresay it's going on all the time. But now you've said no to surgery and will probably go on that weird therapy – has it struck you that if you go through with it, you might become a guinea pig for a lot of people?'

'Frankly, no. I haven't had time lately to think beyond the next step.'

111

'Quite,' said Catherine. 'But you see, if you do go on the therapy and get well, you can then stand on your hind legs and say loud and clear this is what I did, this is what I refused to do, there *is* a choice even with metastasized cancer, and if I could make it, so can others. That would be guinea piggery of a high order. Once you make yourself available as a living example, then a lot of meek and timid people facing their doctors will have the courage to ask questions, make their own decisions and say no, if that feels right to them.'

'Oh, very well. If you put it like that . . . Yes, I suppose the only honest thing is to have a go at the therapy, be my own guinea pig and then say what I feel needs saying. But I can't forgive Lennox and I doubt I ever will.'

Later that day Dr Montague rang to say that the results of the previous day's laboratory tests were largely acceptable, except for my fasting blood glucose which was above normal; he wanted me to go back for a glucose tolerance test. That meant another fast and another frozen early morning trek to the lab, weighed down by weariness. The test turned out to be a ghastly two-hour ritual, starting with a large beaker of sickly, bright yellow glucose drink which made my empty stomach heave; then I had to give blood and pass water half hourly, as instructed by a lugubrious man in a black suit. The experience would have been enough to trigger off any latent Dracula phobia I might have had. The next day Dr Montague informed me that I had mild diabetes. As well.

That came as a shock. It seemed unfair, too, for someone who did not eat sweet things to develop diabetes, as unfair as for a vegetarian to be knocked down by a frozen beef carcase. Even as a child I used to hand round the sweets and chocolates given to me by uninformed adults, a habit that gave me the unearned aura of a saintly, unselfish little girl. The truth was that I could not stand the stuff and much preferred a piece

112

of cheese. And now I had diabetes. I felt much dismayed. But then I realised that this latest twist in my medical saga actually confirmed Dr Gerson's thesis – no cancer without gradually accrued damage to the liver-pancreas system. Obviously my pancreas had degenerated and heaven alone knew what my other organs, especially my liver, were doing. But I pressed on grimly. All day and much of the night I spent every free or sleepless moment reading Gerson's book, in the manner of the frantic pre-exam reading marathons of my student days. I had managed to read a great deal of it by the time I went to visit Margaret Straus on an acrid day in early January.

She lived high up in a block of flats in Bloomsbury. As I approached her flat, I had to bypass a large bag of carrots in order to reach the doorbell. Margaret Straus opened the door. 'You see, we practise what we preach,' she said, shifting the carrots to let me in. She was tall, slim and pretty. She also looked strikingly healthy, with a perfect skin and clear, bright eyes. Just watching her made me aware of how grey, tired and sick I looked.

I told her my story and added that her grandfather's cancer theory had convinced me of the futility of any further orthodox treatment. But where did I go from there, what was I to do?

'Well, you could start on the therapy right away,' she said. 'The treatment is described in full detail in the book, as you know. A lot of patients, not only Jaquie Davison, have recovered by simply following the instructions. I'm not a doctor, I don't examine or treat people in any way. All I can do is to give you practical advice on carrying out the therapy. You'll need a sympathetic doctor to look after the medical side. You've got one? That's excellent; there aren't many around. You'll also have to reorganise your lifestyle and your kitchen. Doing the therapy is a major upheaval, it's difficult and expensive and you'll have to carry on

113

with it for eighteen months or even two years in order to get really well.'

'I gathered that much from Jaquie's story. It's a hell of a long time. Can I work during that period?'

'Not unless you can work at home. You'll have to drink a freshly made raw juice every hour on the hour, so you won't be able to leave the house for any length of time. And at times you'll probably be too weak and ill even to leave your bed, let alone work.'

'In that case I'll lose my job. And my income.'

'I'm afraid I can't advise you on that.'

'No, of course not. Never mind, that's a separate problem. Please tell me more about the practical details of the treatment. I've studied the diet and it looks grim. No doubt you can live on the permitted foods, but don't patients ever die of gastronomic frustration? Eighteen months without an egg or a grain of salt . . .'

'Nobody's ever died of boredom with the diet,' Margaret said. 'But most Gerson patients wouldn't survive long without it. I follow the diet myself out of choice, not necessity, and it's very enjoyable.'

Ah. That explained the large bag of carrots on her doorstep and, probably, her healthy good looks, too. But I still could not imagine how anyone who was not mortally sick could choose to live on that austere ultra-vegetarian regime. However, having been given only six months to live if I refused surgery, I had no business to worry about giving up cucumbers (too salty) or avocados (too oily). Margaret gave me plenty of other topics to worry about. As she explained the routine, I could see that the therapy would reduce my comfortable, free-ranging and sweetly irregular lifestyle to a discipline that smacked of medieval monastic rigour.

There would be no more casual snacks or restaurant meals with friends; I would be restricted to eating at home. All my food would have to be organic, partly to keep poisonous agro-chemicals out of my already heavily toxic system, partly to provide all the vitamins, enzymes, proteins, trace elements and correct sodium-potassium balance that only traditionally grown organic produce contained. That was familiar ground. For some years I had been growing organic herbs and vegetables in my small garden, rather like a modern ecological version of Marie Antoinette pretending to be a milk-maid, and, roughly, with the same impact, since the amounts I produced would have barely fed me for more than a week. Still, I knew the principles. 'Oh good,' said Margaret. 'But you'd need a very large market garden to grow all you need on the therapy.' Indeed, the basic amounts for a week's food and juices were spectacular: thirty-five pounds each of apples and car-rots, twenty pounds of potatoes, ten heads of Cos lettuce, thirty oranges, varying masses of assorted greengroceries from garlic to tomatoes, from celery, beetroot, fennel and onions to green peppers, cour-gettes, sweet corn and radishes. And, of course, extra amounts to feed my helper and any visitors. Margaret told me about the only greengrocer in London who carried a complete organic range and delivered large orders and she hoped that my kitchen was big enough to store a week's supplies. Whatever did not go into juices was to be cooked in purified water, baked in the oven or eaten raw. It sounded dreadfully boring.

Farewell, chopped frozen spinach slowly melting into a velvety béchamel; farewell, tiny tender pale green French peas popping out of tins to cheer me in the depths of winter; adieu, tinned asparagus, tinned everything, good-bye.

Sorry, what was that about purified water? 'Tap water is far too dangerous to drink,' Margaret explained. 'It contains fluoride and chlorine which are enzyme inhib-itors, plus a number of other harmful substances. You either have to install a water distiller which is large and expensive, or buy purified water from the chemist. That's expensive, too, in the long run; you'll need twelve to fourteen gallons a week.'

She allowed me no time to digest the inconvenience of giving up even tap water, as if it were a bad habit, but launched straight into the calamity of the liver, the only non-vegetarian ingredient of the therapy in the shape of three glasses of raw liver and carrot juice a day. The liver had to come from very young calves that had not been exposed to drugs, it had to be fresh, not frozen, and it was fiendishly difficult to obtain. Liver that young lacked taste and was not sold by butchers. Only a few small slaughterhouses could provide it, and even if you found a reliable source, there remained the costly chore of transporting the liver to the patient three times a week.

'That sounds murderously awkward and expensive,' I protested. 'Must I have liver juice? Can't I skip just this one thing?'

'I'm afraid you can't. The liver juice is essential to help restore the patient's sick liver and to supply it with the substances that it can't produce itself for the time being. That's why daily crude liver injections are also part of the programme. At least those aren't difficult to obtain and you can easily learn how to inject yourself. I'd like you to understand that in this therapy every single factor is necessary, nothing can be skipped. It's a total approach; we can't chop it up and skip the awkward parts.'

As she went on, unfolding the details of the therapy that sounded more and more like a full-time job, I realised how lightly I had skimmed over the practical instructions in Gerson's book, concentrating instead on the theory and philosophy of the regime. Well, that was true to form: I had always been one of Nature's own theorists. Except that this time knowing the principles was not enough. Fortunately, my patchy understanding did not put out Margaret. She must have been used to uninformed enquirers. Also, she explained points that were only briefly mentioned in the book, so it was all

116

right for me to admit ignorance. Among them was the business of flare-ups.

'These are favourable reactions to the treatment,' she said. 'They result from rapid detoxification, but they can be much more unpleasant than you'd guess from the book. Pretty foul, in fact. That's one more reason why you need full-time help, someone to look after you during a bad flare-up. Besides, even without flaring you couldn't possibly do all the cooking and juice-making and washing up from morning till night.'

'I'm pretty efficient, you know, and reasonably fit, except for this beastly tiredness.'

She smiled in a way that suggested that I might not stay fit for very long; then she gave me another list of unpleasant details and deprivations. No make-up, no hair colouring, no scent, deodorant or bath oil, no detergents, nothing but plain bland unscented soap for self and laundry, no household or other chemicals, no pressure cooker or aluminium utensils, no push-button juice extractor but a big, heavy electric grinder plus a separate press to squeeze the juice out of the pulped apples and vegetables.

'If I were a militant feminist,' I said, 'I'd suspect the therapy of being anti-woman because it bans all the labour-saving elements of life, from convenience foods to detergents. And to have to make all those juices in two labour-intensive moves – it's really a bit daunting.'

'I know and I'm sorry. But you can't detoxify a poisoned system unless you make sure that it gets no further input of toxic substances, and all the banned things contain harmful stuff. As for centrifugal juicers, unfortunately they produce an exchange of positive and negative electricity that destroys the oxidising enzymes. Yet the sole purpose of the juice therapy is to pour those very enzymes into the body in large quantities. We had some patients who tried to use fast, push-button juicers in order to save time and effort, but they didn't do well at all.'

117

'Oh, very well, I'm grumbling out of ignorance. But frankly, without make-up and hair colouring I'll turn into a grey-haired, sick-looking old thing, and that's no incentive to get well, is it?'

Margaret laughed. 'Ah, but you won't turn into an old thing because as you improve, you'll start looking well and considerably younger, with a good skin and good natural colour. You won't need make-up.'

I shrugged. Much as I liked Margaret, I thought she was far too optimistic. But then – just like Dr Andrews who had also promised me a visible regeneration – she was too young to know that nothing could make good the subtle losses and not so subtle ravages of middle-age. 'Well, I'm afraid I won't give up my eyebrow pencil,' I said firmly and inconsequentially. 'My brows look far too faint without it and my whole face turns wishy-washy. Oh, honestly,' I added, 'aren't I absurd, arguing about my eyebrows when the real subject is my survival? That's the unregenerate female within. Still, I'm glad she's there.'

'I guess it'll be all right for you to keep your eyebrow pencil,' Margaret said with a flicker of amusement.

Shortly afterwards I rose to leave in deep despondency. 'I don't think I can cope with the therapy,' I said sadly. 'I'm ill, I feel terribly weary, I've been through some nasty shocks recently, my house is too small to put up an au pair and it's tough and expensive to get a good daily help. But above all the therapy sounds so complicated and demanding that I don't think I can undertake it. Why isn't there a Gerson clinic somewhere in the world where I could go for a while?'

'But there is one. In Mexico, near Tijuana, just south of the US border.'

'Really? Why didn't you tell me?'

'Because you didn't ask me until now,' Margaret said.

'But I am asking you now! Please go on, tell me more.' Suddenly I felt excited and hopeful once more. If I could start the therapy on the right footing, with

118

expert help, perhaps it would be easier to continue with it at home.

'It's called Hospital La Gloria and it's a very nice place,' Margaret said. 'It's run by a group of doctors who've been trained in the Gerson therapy, and my mother acts as a consultant. If you're interested in going to the clinic, you could ring her tomorrow at her home in California and find out more about the place. Whether they have room for you, and so on.'

'And if I go out, how long would I have to stay?'

'At least three weeks. Obviously the longer you can stay, the better, because the more you learn about the routine, the easier it'll be afterwards at home.'

'Is it terribly expensive?'

It was. In fact, it was as expensive as keeping a patient in a good British hospital. The only difference was that, unlike a stay in a British hospital, the Gerson therapy would not be paid for by the National Health Service.

'Well, well,' I said to Margaret, 'you're certainly not trying to tout for patients. The cost is high. I'd have to use my savings. But then if I die, I shan't need any money and if I get well, I can earn some more. I'd better go away and think about it. Just now it's a bit too much.'

She nodded and compiled a batch of papers for me: a leaflet describing the clinic, the telephone number of her mother, Charlotte Gerson Straus, a selection of recent case histories of Gerson patients newly recovered from so-called incurable conditions, and a stout little booklet on how to pursue the therapy in Britain, complete with useful addresses and special recipes. I clutched the information kit as if it had been the magic thread leading out of the labyrinth. My head felt heavy with facts, fears, doubts, hopes and overwhelming fatigue. I said thank you and good night to Margaret. And I promised to ring her when I had made up my mind. Either way.

119

6

WHEN I GOT home I took the receiver off the hook, lay down on the sofa and drifted off into an unfocussed reverie. I had to find out what I, all of me and not just my brain-box or conscious will, really wanted to do: agree to die of cancer or go on the therapy and try to get well. Both alternatives had become so real in the past few hours that I could imagine either vividly. At the same time my long-lost sense of peace was also beginning to return. There seemed to be nothing left to be tense or anxious about. I had done my market research, inspected the goods and asserted my right to a free choice. All I had to do now was to decide what to buy.

The therapy still sounded exciting – in theory. But the practice, now that I understood its toughness, scared me. Eighteen months of non-life in close confinement, on a programme of all-round deprivation – how could I stick it with my impatient nature and intolerance of boredom? There was an ominous sentence in Dr Gerson's book, under the heading of 'CAUTION – Very Important' which read, 'It is advisable not to start the treatment if for any reason strict adherence to it is not possible.' I had never been good at strict adherence to anything difficult or monotonous and saw little hope of changing now.

But supposing that I did manage strictly to adhere and the treatment still did not work, which was conceivable, would I be furious to have wasted my last few good months, with no strength left to salvage the tail-end and do something truly joyful? For instance, to re-visit some favourite places. Travel now, die later. Design my own last pilgrimage. I would choose a clutch of cathedrals – Chartres, Lincoln, Laon, Vézélay. A string of towns – Bath, Lucca, Trogir, Toledo. Some special spots – Avebury in winter, Painswick in early spring, and in high summer a small hotel in the French Pyrénées with a singing, ecstatic stream rushing past the bedroom windows.

Oh come on, concentrate. The therapy. Yes. If it does not work for me, well, then I will die. Nothing wrong with that. I agreed with Blake's parting words: 'Death is no more than going from one room to another.' Death was as right and as necessary as birth: I had accepted that long ago and did not fear it in the least. Why fear a staging post between two states of consciousness? If I was to die of cancer in the near future, the important thing would be to let go, not cling or struggle, and take leave of the body, slipping away quietly into the next dimension or wherever. Oh, really? a mocking voice asked inside my head; easier said than done. Some years before, when the books of the self-proclaimed Tibetan lama Lobsang Rampa had been all the rage, I had tried very hard to follow his instructions for out-of-the-body astral travel during a grim family occasion when I would have preferred to be anywhere else. But it did not work, my soul had remained firmly wedged inside my body and the experiment turned into an unshareable private joke. Presumably I was far too down-to-earth to leave the physical shell at will. Ah, but terminal cancer might make all the difference.

Sidetracking again. Sorry, sorry. The fact remained that I found it easier to consider the advantages of dying than to drum up enthusiasm for staying alive. It was something to do with the crushing tiredness I felt most of the time, hardly less on waking than at bedtime.

Now in particular, after the breathless chase and emotional tension of the past few days my weariness felt as if nothing short of death might cure it. I thought of an old, battered car I had once seen, its windows plastered with garish stickers proclaiming, 'We've been to Henley' and 'We've been to Cardiff' and so on, all round the country, and one outsize sticker crowning it all with an absolutely final 'We've been everywhere'. No wonder the car had been abandoned in a state of mortal fatigue under a weeping willow in Chiswick. How easy it was to identify with it. Perhaps I, too, had been everywhere without noticing it and there was nowhere else to go.

Death would cure my fatigue. And also the disease of ageing. Whom the gods love die not so much in youth as in middle-age, with a rich track record but no visible sign of decay or deformity. Vanity again. I used to alibi my determination to stay youngish by quoting the example of those courteous old Japanese who dye their hair in order not to depress their friends by reminding them of senescence and mortality, but now that excuse did not work any more. I knew that it was I myself, not my friends, whom I did not wish to depress. I dreaded growing old and ugly. I dreaded the drop in life's temperature, the final loss of intensity. I had always lived in a passionate mode, totally committed to whatever seemed important at any time, so that no experience, good or bad, had been lukewarm or fuzzy. But now, in the nature of things, I could only expect increased middle-aged equanimity and loss of fire, flatness and atrophy, and that was hardly worth living for.

How truly romantic. Or perhaps immature?

This was not getting me anywhere, so I stopped trying to think or decide. A dead friend's self-composed epitaph, 'She loved life and welcomed death', described my situation accurately. There was nothing to add: it was as good as a decision. Now I was slipping into an area where I had to allow meaning to emerge instead of hunting for it, where the opposites of living and dying might become reconciled if not re-balanced. Just now dying had all the best tunes. Lying very still on my blue sofa, I had the impression of swimming fast in a clear, calm sea, free, happy, whole and fulfilled, effortlessly moving farther and farther away from the shore. Oh death where is thy sting? Where, indeed. For death, read freedom.

It was a marvellous timeless moment. And then something strange happened. The hypnotic peace of the experience shattered. So did my detachment. I felt as alert and shocked as if someone had shot me brutally across a vast distance by twanging a rubber band, forcing me back into a dense kind of reality. I must have trespassed into forbidden territory and some invisible frontier guard had kicked me right back where I had come from. But even in my state of shock I knew that what I had sensed about dying and freedom was true and valid; only the timing was inappropriate, and for that reason I would have to go on living.

Serves you right, I thought, for trying to reconcile the opposites out of turn. Being hurled from one extreme to the other was a shock to the system, but also strangely exhilarating. All right, I thought, I will live.

And make something of my life at last, free of the emotional traps and neuroses of my youth and not-so-youth. After all, I had only recently grown proper roots, found aims, begun to round out my pattern. And the people I loved, my precious network of hearts, of love and friendship, suddenly I was overwhelmed by poignant love for them all, for their irreplaceable uniqueness and their warm, zany, ordinary humanity, and I knew I could not bear to leave them. They were part of my pattern, just as I was part of theirs. We were sharing a journey and I had no business to opt out of it unilaterally.

It is up to me, I thought a trifle wildly. It is up to me

whether I live or die, but I have got to make up my mind and stop messing about. If I die now, I will be cheated out of my harvest, my whole life will have been a long preparation with no outcome, a futile exercise. God, I have not done anything yet, only talked endlessly about my plans, and that is not enough. Besides, how hypocritical it would be to reject straight suicide but commit it in mufti, as it were, slowly and by omission.

Above all, how idiotic it would be to die simply because an ignorant surgeon has mismanaged my cancer.

My shock had gone. Now I was angry and full of fight. My repressed resentment towards Mr Lennox and the official cancer establishment exploded into awareness. I went round the house with furious energy and snapped on all the lights. I also opened the windows and the front door to let in the biting January night air. Big deep breaths to fill my lungs. Stretch. Stamp foot. Limber up. Get on with it. Now.

I rang Hudie and told him about my decision. 'I'll go on the Gerson therapy,' I said. 'And I'll start it at the Gerson clinic in Mexico, to learn how it's done properly.'

'Oh, good! I'm so glad. I've been sitting here all evening, worrying my head off and waiting for you to ring. When do you want to leave?'

'As soon as possible. Perhaps early next week. There's no point in waiting while the thing spreads even further. Oh, darling, I hate to leave you, but this is the best way. And I want to stay at the clinic as long as I can afford it. It's expensive.'

'Never mind, I'll help you out. We'll find the money somehow. You've got to get well. You're going to get well, I know it.'

Dear, dear Hudie, with his habitual blind optimism. But this time I managed not to ask 'How do you know?'

and instead said only, 'I hope you're right. If I don't make it, it won't be for lack of trying.'

We said good night. My poor love, I thought, confronted once again with his worst fears, and as they are tied up with me, he cannot even turn round and flee. How will he stand up to the endless months to come, if they come, when he could barely manage those few weeks of my illness a year ago?

It was late, but I quickly rang Catherine to tell her about my decision, and then went to bed with Dr Gerson's book. But this time even the chapter on mineral metabolism in degenerative diseases could not keep me awake for long.

Out of the confusion of dreams that followed, only one fragment survived into waking consciousness. The zodiacal symbol of Scorpio, the sign to which I belong, and the symbol of Cancer were circling and stalking each other on a bleak, rocky shore. Both crustaceans looked deadly and ruthless. They seemed evenly matched, and there was the awesome tension of a life-or-death duel in the way they watched each other's tiniest movement, ready to attack with poisonous sting or crushing pincers.

I could not remember how the dream had ended. Perhaps it had not ended at all, and the fight of the two creatures was continuing at some level and would go on until one of them won and I either got well or died. Well, yes, that made sense. In recent years I had been neglecting the Scorpionic qualities of determination, tenacity and endurance. Perhaps now I would be forced to reclaim them.

7

BECAUSE OF THE time lag between London and California I had to wait until the following afternoon to ring Charlotte Gerson. I felt shaky and shivery as I dialled her number. It frightened me to think that I was trying to arrange a life-or-death matter on the telephone with an unknown lady halfway across the globe. The thought that she might be away or the clinic booked solid for the next year scared me even more.

Charlotte answered at once. I introduced myself, referred to my meeting with her daughter Margaret and asked whether there was room for me at the clinic.

'I don't know off hand, I'll have to check.' She had a clear, crisp voice. 'But first tell me why you want to come.'

'I suffer from malignant melanoma, with a secondary tumour in my groin.'

'Ah well, you'll be glad to know that some of our greatest successes have been with melanoma. One patient whom my father cured twenty-seven years ago is still alive, in the best of health. And we've had many more successes since then. How much surgery have you had?'

'One wide excision, followed by a skin graft.'

'Any radiation or chemotherapy?'

'None.'

'Good. That improves your chances. Some patients who come here have been so badly damaged by ortho-dox treatments that we can't do anything for them. Do you happen to know your current lymphocyte count?'

'Yes, I have the lab report right in front of me. Here we are – lymphocytes thirty-two,' I announced, wondering whether that was good or bad.

'Fine,' said Charlotte. 'It's when the lymphocyte count drops below ten that the therapy doesn't normally work. When was your secondary tumour discovered?'

'Less than a month ago. All I've been offered here is more surgery, which I don't want.'

'Of course not. It wouldn't do you any good. If we have room for you, when could you come?'

'In about ten days' time. Say on the 19th January.'

'Okay, I'm pretty sure we'll be able to put you up one way or another,' Charlotte said cheerfully. 'If you call me again this time tomorrow, I'll be able to tell you more. Meanwhile go ahead and book your flight. You'll have to fly to Los Angeles, change and go on to San Diego, and we'll pick you up from there.'

Nice casual instructions from six thousand miles away, I thought with amusement: that is how I tell first-time visitors how to reach my house from the nearest bus stop. I had no idea how I would arrange everything in such a short time. But from that moment onwards, as if my decision to go ahead had removed an obstacle, everything moved forward smoothly and fast. As in the Irish folk tale, the metaphorical hills flattened themselves and the valleys rose up, allowing me to glide along at speed. Even the discovery that my passport was about to expire did not derail my plans. When I explained at the Passport Office why I had to fly so urgently to the US, the official nodded and said I could collect my new passport two days later.

'You don't give us much time though, do you?' he said gently.

'I'm sorry,' I said. 'I haven't been given much time myself.'

By now I thought I was unshockable, but my new passport photo gave me a jolt. It showed a lifeless, burnt out, totally withdrawn grim face with which I could not identify. But I did not have another picture taken. It would have probably looked even grimmer, since I was feeling worse all the time. The node in my groin felt a little larger every time I touched it. There was also a dull sense of discomfort around my left shoulder blade and armpit.

The next day Charlotte confirmed that there would be a room for me on the 20th, and told me which San Diego motel to stay in after my arrival as it would be too late to transfer me to the clinic that evening. I only paused for a moment to enjoy the good news but did not dare to relax and let go. I was running the show on rapidly shrinking reserves and might not have been able to restart the engine. Please take me through this final spurt, I pleaded inwardly with my body. Please stay the course this last time and forgive my trespasses, including this cigarette and also the next one. If you hold out, poor body, you will be given absolute priority at the clinic. And afterwards. I promise, I promise.

I did not wait for body's reply, but it did not collapse, which was an answer in itself. So I completed a long chain of chores: booked flight, vacated office, collected passport and visas, visited dentist and hairdresser, said goodbye to some friends, wrote to others, picked up dollar cheques and assured my concerned bank manager that I was bloody well going to return from Mexico (in those words, too, shocking the kind man). On top of it all I also started on the Gerson diet as far as possible, which was not very far and consisted mainly in cutting things out. The diet, or the disease, made me lose seven pounds in a week. But as that loss had taken me down to my ideal weight, I refused to worry about it.

Dealing with people who mattered was the hardest task. Trying to convince my weeping mother over the telephone that I would be all right in Mexico, even though no one of our family had ever been there and the Gerson therapy was not exactly world-famous. Trying to explain to my endlessly supportive bosses, Victor and Monica, why the therapy was going to work (and wondering afterwards whether I had been trying to reassure them or myself). Insisting to anxious friends that, yes, I was doing the right thing, yes, I was quite sure, no, I did not want to consult anyone else. Fortunately, there was no need to convince or reassure Catherine when we went for an au revoir meal to a vegetarian restaurant: we talked and behaved as if everything had been normal. At my insistence we rounded off our wholesome, organically grown meal with a large brandy in a raucous pub nearby, as a safeguard against too much virtue. At that stage, for the first time ever, Catherine became oddly protective and urged me to go home by taxi. I refused, but the pub mirror showed me why she was concerned: with my grey face and yellowish eyes I did not look fit enough to walk to the door, let alone travel by public transport.

At some stage during that frantic period I suddenly realised how much Hudie had changed. He was calm, confident and quietly helpful, a strong man ready to take on whatever was coming. There was no trace of the scared small boy, so evident during my previous illness, who had to be shielded from reality. He undertook to set up the therapy in my house in readiness for my return and find someone to do the work. When he explained his plan, I knew with deep gratitude that, barring earthquakes or pestilence, everything would be there and in working order when I came back. I did not know, though, what he really thought about my trip. I myself felt the occasional stab of panic and wondered whether I was completely mad to entrust my life, and most of my savings, to some unknown people in Mexico.

A few days before my departure I rang Ann Procter to thank her for putting me on the track of the Gerson therapy. We had not seen much of each other since finishing our two-year counselling course, but I knew that she worked privately as a healer and teacher of relaxation, and also that she had some cancer patients among her clients. I also remembered her warmth and generosity, and how, during a bakery strike, she had arrived at the course with a basketful of splendid home-baked, wholemeal loaves to help out breadless fellow students. Now, too, she had special nourishment to offer me: if I could make my way to her house outside London, she would teach me the Simonton visualisation technique which she had found a great help with cancer sufferers.

'The technique might be just the thing to take with you to Mexico,' she added. 'Unfortunately, there is nothing in the Gerson therapy to involve the patient's psychological resources in the healing process. Of course, I know that you can work out your own meditation programme, but you might find the Simonton method useful.'

That sounded a good idea. I was on a tight schedule when Hudie drove me out to Ann's house in Surrey. There was not even time to inspect the domestic Mother-Earth side of Ann's life: her beehives, vegetable garden and chicken house. Instead, we went straight to her study and into the Simonton technique. It was simple. Twice a day the patient had to go into deep relaxation and visualise his or her cancer in some symbolic form that sprang spontaneously to mind: as a block of metal, a shark, a science fiction monster or whatever. The next step was to evoke the body's white blood cells, the good guys of the immune system, also in some symbolic shape, and visualise them attacking and destroying the malignant growth. The initial relaxation helped to evoke the images freely. It also dissolved the habitual stresses and tensions which, some researchers now claimed, were cancer-promoting factors. Finally, there was also some goal-setting work, to focus and strengthen the patient's self-confidence and faith in a full recovery – seeing oneself, for instance, as a strong, healthy person, engaged in pleasant activities.

It was good sound stuff, the joint brainchild of an American cancer specialist and his psychotherapist wife, and was based on the powerful link between mind and body, between the will to live and the course of a disease. The Simontons, I gathered, were having remarkable success with cancer patients at their centre in Texas, despite the orthodox treatments those patients had undergone. Clearly, a technique that helped not only against cancer but also against the ravages of conventional therapies had remarkable power.

Thanks to our shared training in the use of imagery, Ann and I were able to sail straight into the exercise, without further preliminaries. The symbol I got for my tumour was a solid black obstruction in a shimmering, colourful internal bodyscape where it sat like a heavy block of negativity. The white blood cells appeared as small, earnest, spherical soldiers wearing bronze helmets and breastplates, looking like members of a comical operatic chorus. They came in orderly waves and attacked the black mass with small bronze swords, chopping and hacking at it but not making much of an impression. *C'est magnifique*, I thought, *mais ce n'est pas la guerre*.

'Don't worry,' Ann said when I reported on my all too tame battle scene. 'You've made a start. The idea is to rally and strengthen the body's defences over a period of time through this symbolic game. You're completely run down and depleted . . . you can't expect a strong response at once!'

'Does the response build up gradually?'

'Yes, it does. The images change all the time and you can tell from the changes how you're doing. For instance, if your white cells first appear as herrings and later turn into swordfish or piranhas, then you know that you're doing well and the process behind the imagery is gaining power.'

131

'I see. And if my piranhas then shrink into toothless goldfish, then I'd better stop and find out what's wrong. I get it. You know, what worries me is the boredom factor – doing the same visualisation twice a day, every day, on top of those endless juices and enemas. It sounds monotonous.'

Ann laughed. 'It *is* monotonous, even though the changing symbols bring in some variety. And you're impatient by nature. It adds up. Haven't you noticed how we regularly fall into beastly situations that hammer away at our weakest points and don't stop until we correct the weakness? It's quite an education.'

'Oh God, yes. The trouble is, I don't feel like being educated just now. It's a bit like the one and only saying of Jung's that always puts my back up – "Freedom of will is the ability to do gladly that which I must do." I've never found that very comforting, but perhaps I'll have to think again.'

Still, that would have to wait, together with further visualisation. On the way home I contemplated the technique. It was sound and logical, but for some reason it left me cold. I did not doubt its validity, only its present relevance to me. I knew that my body was in serious trouble and needed urgent help on the physical level; all else, including psychological back-up, would have to come later. It did not occur to me that the two processes might be combined; I barely had enough strength to deal with one thing at a time.

And then it was time to pack and go. Hudie was unable to see me off on that damp, grey Monday morning; my friend Pat accompanied me to the airport. I was very grateful for her company, for loneliness was closing in on me fast and I urgently needed to be connected to people, above all to my closest friends, but also to strangers, the more the better. If I had had the courage, I would have said to people at large, 'Look, I'm in the position which you all dread, I have cancer, but I'm still a normal human being, not at all different from you except for the way in which some of my cells multiply . . . will you please talk to me and confirm that I still make sense and belong and don't have to be denied?'

I did not say any of this to Pat. There was no need to spell out what I felt. We had a pretty reliable mutual insight into each other's inner states, fuelled by affection and shared experience. Now, on the way to Gatwick we talked as much as ever, laughed less than usual and executed one or two of our ritual skirmishes which we had developed to a fine art over twenty-five years of close friendship. Pat is an agnostic Freudian who enjoys playing Bach, while I am a pan-religious follower of Jung who enjoys listening to Mozart, yet all that these basic differences have ever produced have been hilarious exchanges and occasional concessions to the other's viewpoint. But in the train to Gatwick even our skirmishing was gentler than usual, and I knew that she knew the weight, the deadly weight of that morning, and that she shared it, although her Scottish reserve did not allow her to say so. How was I to express my gratitude to friends beyond price like Pat? Should I perhaps issue a cordial invitation to a celebration at some future date – or to my wake, should things not work out? 'We'll have a party when all this is over,' I mumbled as I hugged her goodbye. Whether I would attend in body or spirit did not have to be specified just then.

An hour or so after take-off I began to enjoy the space and silence of the half-empty aircraft. Space and silence were like a balm. In the past three weeks I had hardly been alone and the lack of privacy had begun to erode me. Off to the ashram, I thought; well, a kind of ashram. The vegetarian meal I had ordered in advance was a stodgy disaster, with an in-flight film to match. It did not matter. Nothing mattered. Far below, the world looked empty and endless. First the empty endless sea, then the endless flat white emptiness of Canada, so vast and desolate. It was strange to find so much empty space left on this earth. Then sleep, empty flat white sleep.

By the time I arrived in San Diego via the diabolical airport of Los Angeles, it was three in the morning by my body-clock against the local time of eight pm. The motel I had been booked into was clean, cheap and totally without service of any kind. There was no food, no drink, no one even to carry my suitcase up the staircase. I found I did not have the strength to take it up myself, which frightened me, because normally I could lug around quite heavy loads. In the end a kind fellow guest hauled up my bag. I was starving but could not face going out in search of food. The thing to do (I remembered this from a broadcast by the explorer Wilfred Thesiger) was to lie flat on my stomach until the hunger pangs ceased.

But first I rang the Gerson Institute. A man answered. I confirmed that I had arrived, he confirmed that I would be picked up at ten in the morning. That was that. Then I fell asleep.

8

IT TOOK ME a while to wake up properly in that weird motel room with its jokey notices from the management (but no breakfast, no plug for the hand basin, no handles on the drawers). The place felt unreal and so did I. No one close to me knew exactly where I was and this made me feel out of context. I touched my groin gingerly – perhaps crossing an ocean and a continent had made the lump vanish? But no, it was there, feeling bigger still. Was it growing a little every day? If it was, where would it stop? Ah, the therapy, of course, that was going to stop it, that was what I was here for. Through my jet lag things were slowly swimming into focus. I got up and looked out of the widow, right across the hazy blue of San Diego harbour. Ah, the Pacific, I thought stupidly. But I was too hungry to savour that first glimpse.

I got dressed and went in search of food. The nearest hotel was bustling with convention delegates, but I soon got into the coffee shop and ordered the biggest breakfast on the menu. The waitress brought a big bowl of fresh fruit – pineapple, slices of honeydew and water melon, an apple, grapes, an orange, a banana, lychees, a nectarine, all the glory of California's orchards. And I ate the lot, doggedly and with joy. Then came two large cups of coffee and four slices of delicate toast with lashings of butter, marmalade and honey, each mouthful eaten with the passion of a convicted prisoner enjoying a last meal in the death cell. When I could not swallow another mouthful, I lit a cigarette. The woman

135

at the next table screwed up her face and waved at my smoke which was actually curling away from her; she was letting me know that I was a nasty anti-social air polluter, but I simply looked away.

Too bad, sister, I thought. Sorry to upset you, but I am smoking my last cigarette for a very long time, if not for the rest of my life. It is my only addiction and I have no idea how I will manage without it, having smoked since the age of nineteen with only brief breaks whenever I thought I could give it up. And every time I realised that I could not, the shame of yet another broken resolution was cancelled out by the pleasure of lighting up and being comforted, rather like going back to an evil lover who would probably kill me in the end but was indispensable in the meantime. And so (I continued with my inner monologue) I am going to smoke this one to the end, and God alone knows how I am going to cope with the therapy and the strains and stresses of my dicey situation without cigarettes. At least Mr Lennox never told me to stop smoking (and look where that has landed you, my more sensible inner voice cut in).

On the way back to the motel I dropped my cigarettes and matches into a dustbin and walked on, feeling bereft and heroic. But back in the motel room I just felt stupid. I could have had another soothing smoke while waiting to be picked up. I experienced the familiar panic of countless late nights in the past when I had stubbed out my last cigarette, knowing that I could not possibly get another pack until the morning; but now this *was* the morning and there would not be another one ever again, amen. God, what a weak, pathetic, panicky, dummy-craving creature I was. Amen, amen.

The clinic's minibus arrived and the young driver escorted me downstairs. There were three passengers in the bus: a tall, pale, angular young Dane by the name of Mike who announced that he had melanoma as if that had been part of the information people normally

136

gave when introducing themselves, and an elegant middle-aged woman, Becky, from Baltimore, accompanied by her daughter Sally. I sat next to Becky. She had an intelligent, humorous face with warm brown eyes. She also had, she informed me, metastasized lung cancer, following two radical mastectomies. The way she said this, in a calm, vaguely apologetic voice, made her statement even more shattering. Compared to her trouble, my massacred leg and solitary lump sounded almost harmless. I said so, too, as I introduced myself, but Mike disagreed.

'Don't underestimate melanoma,' he said. 'It's a real devil. It may not sound bad, but once it takes off, you can't stop it. I've been to several unorthodox clinics with mine when I discovered that the doctors couldn't do anything for me. I've already been to the Gerson clinic, too, and I did quite well but afterwards I couldn't keep up the therapy in Canada where I live. Couldn't get organic vegetables, couldn't get the right kind of liver. So I'm back again, and I just hope that this time I'll get well, because there's nowhere else to go.'

I did not like that. I did not like Mike, either. He seemed utterly negative, his hair not so much blond as drained of colour, his voice creaky dry, his young face already creased by habitual disapproval. Yet while disliking him I also wanted him to improve, to get cured. He was the first of several melanoma patients who made me feel that way. Our shared disease created an instant bond between us, and if one of us got well on the therapy, there was hope for the others, too.

We were driving through well-groomed Southern Californian suburbs with luxuriant greenery, flowering shrubs and impeccable, over-pretty houses. As soon as we crossed the border into Mexico – the Mexican frontier guards showed no interest in the US-registered cars streaming past them – the greenery stopped abruptly and dust and disorder took its place. We

137

passed a huge road-building project and the large, half-finished concrete shells of future supermarkets and offices, but all this mega-activity was taking place in a beige desert, unrelated to anything else.

'You'll enjoy your stay at the clinic,' the driver said. 'It's an unusual place, kind of inspiring. Some really fine people there. If you don't speak Spanish, you'll have some communication problems . . . only Mexicans can be employed at the clinic, that's the law here, and the maids and nurses speak very little English or none. The doctors do, of course. Just use sign language with most of the staff. They're friendly and kind girls. If you show them respect and don't try to rush them, you'll be okay.'

The wide, dusty road was lined with second-hand car showrooms, garages, parking lots fringed with clapped-out flashy American cars labelled FOR SALE, more garages, repair shops, and nothing else. 'It's the Mexican petrol,' the driver explained. 'The stuff is very hard on the engine. That's why there's such a high turnover in used cars.' Ugliness everywhere. My heart sank. Across the road, clusters of makeshift hovels were clinging to the hillside, festooned with washing lines. All right, I was not here for the sightseeing, but was this the only face of Mexico I was going to meet? I recognised the ugliness of the typical borderland, made worse here by the meeting of wealth and poverty: those destitute Mexicans in their cardboard and plastic hovels were probably straining towards the US as illegal immigrants, while the worst of the American way of life – car mania, concrete deserts, consumerism – was washing southbound across the border. Sad, sad. I abandoned the Mexican imagery I had brought with me of the hibiscus, the white-washed adobe houses, the patient donkeys and the high peaks, and decided to suspend all expectations.

A vivid clump of greenery appeared on the right. The driver swung the car off the road, through a wide gate into the forecourt of La Gloria Hospital, the home of the Gerson clinic. He stopped outside two long, low, single-storey buildings separated by a narrow open passage. Beyond that a flight of steps and a steep path led up the hillside towards a larger two-storey structure. Halfway between the two, where the path veered left, there stood a cosy-looking brown cottage with a terrace. And all over the grounds the luxuriant palms, cacti, agaves and glossy evergreen trees looked well-tended and plump with moisture. After the deadly aridity outside it was good to know that my gardener's eyes would have some living, growing things to feast on. The place looked pleasantly informal, unlike any hospital I had ever seen.

Becky, her daughter Sally, Mike and I stood around with the awkwardness of newcomers until a plump nurse with gold teeth bade us to sit down in the mild January sunshine. It was a balmy, lukewarm day, a whole season ahead of the cities the four of us had come from, and we sat basking in the bright light, admiring the colourful Mexican toy animals Sally had bought for her small sons. It had been Sally's idea to bring Becky to Mexico when her lung cancer had been diagnosed. Her brother, Becky's elder son, had championed orthodox treatment for their mother, but Sally, whose face was as strong and wild as Becky's was meek and compliant, had fought him off and driven her mother south of the border. Becky's scientist husband, I gathered, had been too upset to take part in the family debate.

'There are quite a few unorthodox cancer clinics in this area, around Tijuana,' Becky said. 'We drove around and visited a few. At first I wanted to go to Dr Contreras's clinic; he's supposed to be a marvellous man and he uses Laetrile with some success. But he wasn't there, and I liked the atmosphere of this place so much that I decided to come here instead.' She sat in a curiously contorted way, hugging the back of the chair, her legs crossed and twisted round the chair-leg. It was the typical unrelaxed posture of someone who constantly expects to have to jump up and wait on others, guess unspoken needs and clear away after everybody.

A youngish man with perfect Inca features appeared, introduced himself as Dr Vic, welcomed us and disappeared. Nurses came and went; also some people, wearing unmistakably American leisure clothes, who, I presumed, were patients' relatives or visitors. (It took me a day or two to realise that most of them were patients, and that it was a general rule to be up and about, walk in the grounds and eat in the dining-room whenever possible.) There was only one obviously sick person in view, a stubble-chinned, terribly emaciated young man, pushed along in a wheelchair by a pretty but burstingly fat girl.

Eventually we were called to the administrator's office to register and receive our information folder and a copy of Dr Gerson's book – *the* book, as we all referred to it – which was our only source of information and, through the case histories, of hope. Then a handsome Mexican boy, Marcos Aurelios, took my baggage to my quarters. I was to stay in the brown cottage which contained two apartments; mine was the one with the sun terrace which, I now noticed, was covered with green plastic grass carpet. Marcos Aurelios spoke some English and often frowned in a concentrated, manly fashion that promised – quite falsely, as I later discovered – efficiency and prompt attention.

As the door closed behind him, I sat down on the bed and looked around. The room was modestly furnished, in the style of a drab hotel room, refreshingly un-hospital-like. There was nothing of visual interest, except a large colour photo of two over-cute kittens above the bed. A hard couch, covered in brown plastic, stood opposite the bed; at one end a wrought iron pole with curly hooks on either side rose from the wooden frame. I concluded that this must be the enema couch. In the bathroom a notice pleaded for a sparing use of water, as we were in a drought-stricken zone. That referred to bathing and flushing only. For all other purposes there was a huge bottle of purified water standing in the corner.

I thought of Hudie and of my comfortable house in London and was just about to turn despondent when there was a knock on the door. 'Jews!' a voice called outside. Then a hefty maid entered, carrying a trayful of khaki-coloured drinks in tall glasses. 'Jews!' she repeated, handing me a glass. Ah, juice, I thought, identifying the word I was to hear thirteen times a day for the next two months. Sometimes it was augmented to 'More Jews!' by girls who liked to show off their vocabulary. It was noon, so this had to be a green drink, despite its beige-olive colouring. I took a sip. What hit my taste buds was a strong, earthy, complex flavour, both sweet and tart; above all, strangely alive in its freshness, quite unlike any juice I had ever tasted. The relevant list in my information folder told me that I was drinking a blend of apple, Cos lettuce, green pepper, red cabbage, sprouted seeds, watercress and wheat-grass. It was not bad; as long as the others were not worse.

I looked at the information folder. The hourly sched-ule for Gerson patients looked horrendous. It stretched from eight in the morning to seven in the evening and set out the day's duties. The first column gave the correct order of the hourly juices. Orange, green, apple and carrot, liver, green, apple and carrot, green, liver, liver, apple and carrot, apple and carrot, green, apple and carrot, I read down the column. At half a pint each that added up to six and a half pints a day – a hell of a lot of juice. Then came seven columns of medication, to be taken at various times throughout the day: Acidoll Pepsin capsules, potassium compounds solution, Lugol half-strength solution, thyroid, niacin and pancreatin tablets, and crude liver injections laced with vitamin B 12. At least these were natural substances, not synthetic drugs. Then came the coffee enemas, 'every four hours or more as needed', I read with a shudder; plus castor oil treatment 'every other day'. Cause for a strong shudder. Oh, well, that is what I had come for. Shudder and be cured.

The next leaflet explained the correct way to sprout seeds such as alfalfa, lentils, chick peas, wheat and beans. There was nothing new or threatening about that. I had long been growing and eating these sprouts, though somewhat irregularly, as a perfect supply of fresh natural vitamins and minerals. In future, I would have to sprout seeds regularly. The next piece of information, on how to inject oneself with crude liver or whatever, looked weird: it depicted a man's hand spread out over somebody's bare hip, with the hipbone mysteriously showing through body and hand. But it was all right, we were being shown how to find the correct spot for the needle in the ventrogluteal site. Alas, from another drawing I could also see how an inexperienced operator like myself could stick the needle, without any difficulty, straight into the sciatic nerve, causing vile pain and bother. I did not care for that possibility, so I looked at the recipe booklet instead. There was nothing inspiring about that, either. Vegetables were to be cooked slowly and at length with minimal water, or on a bed of chopped tomatoes or apples to provide moisture. Ugh. But then nobody promised me a Cordon Bleu diet. Perhaps it was best not to read too many recipes in one sitting.

Shortly before one o'clock I went to the dining-room in the administrative block. The décor was friendly and bland, with a mock-rustic chimney piece and a disused cocktail bar. Above the fireplace there hung a photograph of Dr Gerson. I studied it at length, realising that until that moment I had not even tried to imagine what he had looked like. Now I saw a keenly intelligent face

142

with a high forehead and observant eyes, an archetypal doctor's face of the kind I had known as a child: gentle, wise and understanding, but with a firm streak, the face of a man who made you feel better simply by listening to what you had to say.

'Don't you wish Dr Gerson were alive?' a man's voice asked behind me. 'I did, until I realised that even if he were alive, he'd be a hundred years old and long retired. I guess we'll have to get on without him. My name's Carl, I'm from Atlanta, Georgia. Who are you?'

His rich Southern accent threw me for a moment. I thought he had said his name was Coral – could that be a nickname on account of his colouring? He had curly ginger (or was it coral red?) hair, topped with a wildly clashing cherry-red jockey cap. Underneath his curly ginger beard a black T-shirt proclaimed in glittering script, 'I LIKE MONEY, CHAMPAGNE, CADILLACS'. The effect was totally disarming. But Coral? Ah, it must be Carl, I thought, and introduced myself.

Carl scrutinised me. 'I'll call you Bee,' he decided. 'It's simpler. What's your problem?'

As I was to discover, that question was the standard conversation opener among patients at the clinic. Most people had advanced cancer and most of them discussed their illnesses freely, without the usual euphemisms and deathly hushed tones. Their general openness made the atmosphere so light and confident that sufferers from other diseases, such as multiple sclerosis or crippling rheumatoid arthritis tended to explain almost apologetically that they did not, in fact, have cancer. But there were some who preferred not to talk about their 'problem', and that was immediately accepted. I decided, gladly, to be open.

'My problem,' I said, 'is malignant melanoma, with a secondary tumour in my right groin. What's yours?'

Carl grinned. 'Mine's exactly the same! Well, well. We must stick together. I know this place quite well, I'll be glad to assist you until you learn the ropes. At first it's pretty bewildering.'

The dining-room was filling up. A beautiful old lady with an ominous rash on her face made a regal entrance. Nobody else was visibly marked, everyone looked lively. A thin, elderly man staggered in, bent double with laughter. 'That's Ed,' Carl explained. 'He enjoys his own jokes so much that we all have to laugh, even though half the time we don't know what it's about.' The beautiful old lady was Emily, he added in a low voice. She was over eighty and her rash was cancerous, but she was battling on. At that stage Becky and Sally joined us and we sat down at a table for four, ready for a genuine Gerson lunch.

There was a jug with lemon-and-water salad dressing on the table, a bottle of linseed oil and a plateful of peeled raw cloves of garlic, flanked by a garlic press. Garlic, I recalled, was reputed to have anti-cancer properties, and cancer incidence was low in those areas of southern Europe where garlic consumption was high. It was just as well I liked the stuff. There was, of course, no salt or pepper on the table.

A maid brought a huge bowl of mixed salad for our first course. Lettuce, frizzy endive, tomatoes, spring onions, radishes, all crisp and young. Another girl handed out large glasses of brilliant yellow carrot and apple juice. I sipped mine and found it curiously thick and tasty. (No other carrots I have tried since – English, French or German – were remotely as creamy and fragrant as those Californian ones. On the Gerson therapy you become a true connoisseur of carrots.)

Next, a pink plastic medicine box with six labelled compartments landed in front of me. 'Take the medication marked 1 pm,' said the nurse who had brought it. 'Start with the two capsules and leave the tablet with the line across it until after you've finished your meal. Please do the same,' she told Becky, handing her a similar blue medicine container.

'I'm almost sure to take them in the wrong order,' Becky admitted, examining her 1 pm portion of medicines, two capsules and five tablets in all. 'This kind of straightforward instruction makes my mind seize up at once.'

'Don't worry, it's simple when you know why the order is important,' Carl said. 'The capsules come first because they aid digestion. The plain white tablets, thyroid and pancreatin, are taken while you eat. But the niacin or nicotinic acid – that's the one with the line across it – comes last, when you've finished eating. If you take it with food or drink, you may get a violent reaction which makes you turn dark red and very hot, as if you were running a high temperature. It's harmless and doesn't last long, but you might just as well avoid it.'

Becky and I nodded solemnly. It was just like learning the rules in a new boarding school. To cheer us up, Carl told us the story of one of Dr Gerson's early melanoma patients which served as a cautionary tale at the clinic. Apparently, way back in 1954, this man was improving rapidly on the therapy when he experienced his first red-hot niacin reaction. Not having been prepared for it, and being of a religious bent, he mistook it for a divine omen signalling his miraculous recovery. Or, more accurately, he thought that the prickly redness and heat flooding his skin equalled the allergic inflammation which, in Dr Gerson's view, was vital in the healing process. So he abandoned the strict diet and shortly afterwards suffered a relapse. Dr Gerson promptly put him back on the strict therapy for another fourteen months, after which the patient recovered. 'He's still around,' Carl concluded. 'He's a big, strong guy, full of pep. You may meet him, he drops in sometimes to encourage us.'

We ate large portions of salad with some sharp dressing but no linseed oil. Our daily oil ration was only two tablespoons and we would need all that to

145

cheer up the saltless baked potatoes. The dietary mercies, I observed, were very small.

After the salad came the special soup, prescribed by Hippocrates around 550 BC as a detoxifying substance for cancer sufferers and rediscovered by Dr Gerson in 1928. It was thick enough to eat with a fork and was the very essence of humble vegetables: onions, leeks, celeriac, potatoes, parsley root and tomatoes, cooked in water and milled into a velvety pink-beige purée. It had enough natural flavour not to need salt or spices. Following Carl's lead, I squeezed a raw garlic clove through the press into the soup. The result was powerful.

'I like the soup,' Becky said after a while. 'It's comforting.'

'You'd better like it a lot,' Carl warned, 'because you'll have it twice a day every day for a long time. Except somehow it always tastes slightly different.'

The main course consisted of a large baked potato, which we garnished with cold linseed oil and more raw garlic, and a helping of broccoli. Finally, we had some fresh fruit. My doubts began to whisper again. This was a good vegetarian wholefood meal, I thought, minus fat or seasoning, but unsensational; could such an elementary diet really work against cancer? The conversation from the other tables washed over me. This was my chance to study regional accents from various parts of the US. I could already understand almost everything Carl was saying in his thick southern drawl.

Hardly had I lain down in my room for a rest when another large green juice arrived, and I had to accommodate it somehow on top of my ample lunch. Those hourly juices, each one half a pint of sparkling liquid nourishment, were quite a shock at first. I recapitulated the theory behind them. The depleted body had to be bombarded at short and regular intervals with the live vitamins, minerals and oxidising enzymes contained in the juices; only in juice form could the necessary huge amounts be taken and absorbed. That much was clear. But in practice, by the end of that first afternoon, after two glasses of carrot and liver juice, another green and three more apple and carrot juices, my stomach felt rebellious. Was I being flooded or flushed, doused or drowned? Was I afloat or abloat, and would I eventually burst?

Between the two liver and carrot juices at three and four in the afternoon (curiously enough they tasted of slightly peculiar tomato juice), I lay on my bed, waiting for the worst part of the therapy to materialise. When it did, it had the additional drawback of being presented by Marcos Aurelios who arrived with two plastic enema buckets in sealed bags, and a large jug of coffee.

'I show you how to have enema,' he declared.

'Oh no, you don't. I want a nurse to teach me.'

'I am a nurse,' he said with hurt dignity.

'Perhaps you are, but I want a female nurse, please. A girl,' I added, to make myself quite clear. Marcos Aurelios frowned and shook his head. No doubt from where he sat, on the fence of his seventeen years, it seemed odd that an ancient lady like myself should mind whether her first enema was administered by a male or a female nurse. But he did go away in a sulk, and shortly afterwards a lovely Mexican girl arrived, all dressed in snowy white summer clothes, with a superbly embroidered white cape around her shoulders. She looked dazzling, bridal and totally incongruous. I suspected that she was a nurse whom Marcos Aurelios had caught between two shifts. I pointed at her cape and said, 'That's really beautiful.'

'Ah! Acapulco,' she replied, interpreting my gesture, for she spoke no English. But she rewarded me with a pirouette to show off her cape, and a big smile. Then she initiated me slowly and carefuly into the preparation of the coffee enema, using sign language and demonstration to specify the correct quantity of coffee and the right temperature of water. She also assisted me in my first effort to take it. It was awkward, slightly unpleasant and bizarre, and the process revived childhood memories, because when I was small and my metabolism sometimes failed to function with the precision of a fine Swiss watch, my mother would haul me off to the bathroom and administer a corrective enema. Of mildly soapy water, of course, not one part of coffee to three of water. The sensation had not become more pleasant since then, but now, as then, I had no choice.

All this flashed through my mind while my glamorous all-white instructress floated over me and the deep brown couch like a luminous angel, providing a vivid contrast to the dark goings-on. Obviously she found the whole business perfectly ordinary and patted me on the shoulder by way of farewell. She also said something in Spanish which I interpreted as 'Don't worry, you'll get used to it.'

No doubt, no doubt. But the prospect of five or even six such operations a day, each taking around twenty-five minutes, was awesome. I picked up the book and re-read the relevant passage to convince myself that there was no alternative, and discovered that things could be even worse when I found this: 'In the beginning . . . on the average we give coffee enemas every four hours, day and night, and even more frequently against severe pain, nausea, general nervous tension and depression.' Hold it, I thought, I do not suffer from any of those afflictions, and besides, with all due respect, if my soul aches, filling my colon with coffee and water is not likely to help much. But then the word 'detoxification' leapt off the page and straight into my consciousness, and I stopped arguing. Like a schoolchild trying to memorise unfamiliar new material, I tested my memory to see if I knew why coffee enemas were necessary. Let me see. The caffeine was absorbed from the colon through the haemorrhoidal and portal veins into the liver and stimulated the production of bile which then flowed more freely, speeding up the elimination of toxins from the liver. Did I get it right? Yes, I did, according to page 191.

I went on to read another paragraph: 'More advanced cases are severely intoxicated and the absorption of the tumour masses, glands, etc., intoxicates them even more. Many years ago I lost several patients by coma hepaticum (coma of the liver), since I did not know, and therefore neglected, the vital importance of frequent and regularly continued elimination of poisonous substances with the help of juices, enemas, etc.'

Lovely man, Dr Gerson, I thought; admits in print that he lost patients through his ignorance. Doctors are supposed to bury their mistakes discreetly, not confess them in public, but he is – was – different. He gives no instructions, either, without explaining the reasoning behind them. 'Patients have to know,' I read on the same page, 'that the coffee enemas are not given for the function of the intestines but for the stimulation of the liver.' Yes, Doctor, this patient knows it.

But even so, with full understanding, it was uncomfortable to have to confront and concentrate on the unknown processes within my belly and on my equally unknown, unimagined digestive organs. How odd to acknowledge having portal veins (what were they, anyway?), large stores of toxins in my liver, and miles, or was it yards, of convoluted guts, all of this belonging to my digestive underworld that felt as remote and mysterious as the original Greek Hades. It was an underworld, too; a dark and denied area with its invisible operations and strange, muffled sounds that are not discussed except by way of joking or swearing, both modes being emotion-laden and inaccurate. What is more, that underworld was the physical equivalent of the unconscious that was also habitually denied and kept out of sight until it rebelled and took revenge. From my rich hoard of useless information there popped up the term 'borborygmus', the medical term for rumbling guts – and also the old Greek word for the

149

filth and mud of Hades. There was a fascinating parallel here between myth and physiology, guts and psyche that I urgently wanted to discuss with Catherine. But the impulse wilted when I remembered where I was and that there would be no discussions with her, or anyone else in London, for a long time.

So I went on pondering some basics on my own. For instance, in our society, to consume is all right and praiseworthy, to excrete is not, so that the function has to be hidden behind the strictly clinical or behind pastel-pretty bathroom fittings with matching loo paper and air fresheners. In the latter case excretion itself turns into a form of consumption. There is not much balance here, I thought, no respect for the vital cycle of input and output (which every compost-making gardener understands). Little wonder we have become such a toxic society, absorbing poisons from all sides but giving no thought to getting rid of them.

This speculation was interrupted by yet another juice and immediately afterwards by the arrival of a tall, young Mexican woman doctor, called Dr Elsa, who had come to examine me. She carried out an incredibly thorough examination, the most searching I had ever had. Halfway through it I felt that most of my cells must have been inspected, turned inside out and checked, and still the questions kept coming. The only question she did not ask was the one that had interested Mr Lennox to the exclusion of all others – whether I had ever lived in a tropical climate. But then here my melanoma would not have been ascribed to too much sunshine or other external factors.

Towards the end of the examination I asked Dr Elsa what treatment I would get for my newly discovered diabetes.

'None,' she answered. 'You need no specific treatment. Your diabetes will go.'

'Do you mean it'll go spontaneously?'

'Oh yes, the therapy will clear it up as you go along.

Don't forget, this is a non-specific therapy that heals the whole organism, so you need no special treatment for your diabetes.'

Oh yes, of course. I just hoped she was right.

'Please make sure you don't miss a single enema,' Dr Elsa said. 'That's entirely your responsibility. No one will check how many you take a day. But don't skip any, especially during a flare-up. That's when detoxification is vital.'

'When do patients normally start having flare-ups?'

'It varies. Some start almost at once, others take a while. There's no rule.'

When she had left I wanted to rest, but another juice arrived, and I also realised that there was just enough time for an enema before dinner. All this busyness was bewildering. You had to be quite fit just to keep up with the schedule. The day was almost over and I had not even been able to unpack, let alone rest or sleep or explore La Gloria or, indeed, meditate. And to do the latter had been one of my top priorities.

My mouth tasted odd. I inspected my tongue in the bathroom mirror and found that it was heavily brown-coated. Fast work, I thought. My body is already unloading toxins after only six hours on this weird regime.

'Sure they keep you busy here,' Carl said at dinner when I commented on the crowded timetable. 'And you've only seen half of it. Every morning there's a lecture on some aspect of the therapy which we're expected to record for future reference. That's why you had to bring your cassette recorder all the way from home. We're also supposed to spend some time in the kitchen and watch how the juices are made. Then there's a talk by Charlotte Gerson every Saturday afternoon. By the time we leave here we'll really know how to run the therapy.'

Carl himself had no plans to leave. His private insurance policy covered his stay for a long period, and although he admitted that living at La Gloria felt monotonous and isolating, he preferred to stay put. 'I tried to do the therapy at my parents' house after my first stay here two months ago,' he said, 'but it was hellishly difficult and my tumour started to grow again. So I came back here and I won't leave until my eighteen months are up. Unless my insurance firm goes bust first.'

'Eighteen months!' Becky exclaimed. 'I can only stay for two weeks and even that seems a long time.'

'But you need at least three weeks here, not two,' Carl said.

'Well, you see, I've got to look after my husband,' Becky explained with a small nervous smile. 'And there's my mother, too. She lives in our vicinity and can't do her own shopping, I have to do it for her, so I really must get back soon and . . .'

'Oh, yeah?' Carl cut in. 'And if you don't get well, who's going to look after them? Who's going to look after *you* when you go home, eh?'

'I'll sort that out later. There's always a solution,' Becky said. She was on the defensive and kept smiling, not wanting to upset Carl. Did she ever allow herself to upset anyone, or was she one of those self-effacing, peace-at-any-price good women who inevitably end up as victims? But it was not the right moment to discover more about her. At the end of the meal some people joined us from neighbouring tables to find out who Becky and I were, and where we came from. Becky got away lightly – Baltimore was not exotic enough to inspire many questions. I, however, had to go through the usual London, England routine with those friendly, curious Americans who had either been in London, England, or were planning to visit it by way of celebration when they had completed the therapy and were well again. It was always when, not if. That first evening I picked up the prevailing mood of patients that largely remained the same throughout my two

152

months in Mexico: a mood of hope, cautious optimism and determination to get well. The odd patient who sometimes became depressed or fearful was quickly boosted or ticked off by a fellow sufferer. Despondency was resented and discouraged, as if we had all been linked by a net of collective consciousness through which any one person's fear or despair communicated itself to everyone else and had to be tackled fast.

Emily, the beautiful old lady with the cancerous rash around her nose and eye, sat down next to me. 'I want to live to be a hundred,' she declared. 'I'm eighty-one and there are still a lot of things I want to do in this life.'

'If you want it badly enough, you'll do it all,' Carl said. 'But you'll have to stick to the diet forever.'

'Oh, I know that!' The old lady turned to me. 'My dear, I used to live in France. Now I'm paying the price of forty years of rich French food . . . it was glorious, but it ruined my digestion. So I can't really object to this diet.' She had limpid brown eyes and a delicate nose that looked as if it had been skilfully stitched together.

Two young girls, identical twins, passed our table with their mother. 'We're going home tomorrow!' one of the girls shouted. 'See you at breakfast!' No, they did not have straightforward cancer, Carl explained, they suffered from a malignant type of arterial trouble, the so-called pulseless disease. But they were improving rapidly.

'Is everybody here improving rapidly?' I asked. 'It sounds almost too good.'

'No, some of us are just holding our own,' a tall black woman, whom I had not noticed before, said quietly. 'But that's more than what we'd do elsewhere.' Her name was Doris. She was a highly trained nurse, so experienced that when her breast cancer had been diagnosed, she had refused orthodox treatment and travelled to Mexico instead. She had a deep, amused voice and great dignity. 'Excuse me, it's time for my coffee break,' she said and left the dining-room. That, I discovered, was one of the local euphemisms for having an enema, together with upside-down coffee or, simply, being busy. Patients engaged in that vital part of the therapy locked their doors and lowered their blinds to indicate that they were not to be disturbed. When they mis-timed their coffee breaks so that the tray-bearing hourly maids could not hand over their juices, there was some mutual shouting through locked doors – shouts of 'Jews! Jews!' countered with 'Ah'm having a coffee break!' in varying tones of apology or despair. In such cases the glasses of juice, covered with foil caps, were left on our window sills and had to be rescued and drunk as soon as possible, since those all-important enzymes deteriorated fast.

At nine o'clock, after a bothersome final enema, I went to bed feeling peaceful and passive. Watching the ceiling was quite satisfactory – I did not want to read, write or even think. Yes, the room needed a coat of paint and something resembling a colour scheme, and the blankets were too thin and I felt a million miles away from my own world, but despite all that I knew I was in the right place and my body felt extraordinarily relaxed and comfortable. By the time I registered my sense of well-being I was more than half asleep.

9

ALL MY LIFE I have needed silence and privacy first thing in the morning, to help me over the pain of waking up from the deep-sea satisfaction of sleep. At La Gloria, however, this old weakness of mine was cured at a stroke: there was simply no time to feel the agony of rising from the ashes, no time to meditate, do some yoga or gaze at the dawn sky, waiting for the bio-rhythms to adjust to daylight. Instead, I had to snap into wakefulness at the first pip of my alarm clock – getting up at the right time was the patient's responsibility – and immediately proceed to the enema couch; and that was no place for gentle reverie or contemplation.

In theory that first descent into the underworld should have taken place at six o'clock, so that by repeating the performance every four hours patients could complete the day's enema quota by ten in the evening, except the very sick who also needed a 2 am repeat. In practice I cheated and did not start until seven. Even that seemed absurdly early. Instead of lifting up my spirit to the peaks – or, better still, leaving it well alone – I had to lower my attention to my darkest inner space, amid much discomfort and some resentment. It was most certainly a strange way to start the day.

Barely had I crept back to bed when a young Mexican nurse arrived. She was thin, short and earnest and walked with the stiff gait of a clockwork maiden. Her name, she whispered, was Alberta. She had tiny, gentle hands, and her lack of English caused no problem while she took my temperature, pulse and blood pressure and then prepared to administer a crude liver injection. It was only after she had stuck the needle into my flank that she spoke, timidly uttering the single word, 'Penn?' I heard the question-mark in her voice but she had to repeat the word three times before I understood that she was asking whether I was suffering pain. On subsequent mornings I tried to teach her to ask 'Does it hurt?' and for a while seemed to succeed, but then 'penn' returned and I let it be. Despite the linguistic hurdles Alberta and I enjoyed a good relationship.

Breakfast came at eight: a large tumbler of freshly pressed orange juice, a bowl of saltless, milkless porridge, a bowl of stewed dried fruit and a banana. There was also the medication out of my refilled pink plastic box which was bursting with thirty tablets, capsules and pills, to be taken in six instalments throughout the day. Like so much else, swallowing the right medication at the right time was also my responsibility. Following the Gerson timetable was like travelling on a non-stop express train, being both passenger and driver.

Well, all right, let me try and enjoy the trip. I got dressed and moved out into the sweet sunshine and mild breeze of the morning. It was supposed to be the rainy season, but the only moisture in sight came from a gardener's hose. The path was edged with pretty yellow and purple flowers that might have been daisies except for their fleshy succulent leaves. I sat down on the sun terrace and basked in the morning radiance. At rest, at last.

Not for long, though. At nine the green juice arrived, followed by Becky who wanted to know how on earth we were supposed to manage the ten o'clock red juice, the ten o'clock enema, the ten-fifteen castor oil and the eleven o'clock lecture. 'It can't be done,' we exclaimed simultaneously and burst out laughing, but Becky began to cough and then, gasping for air, tried to

156

apologise. 'Please don't, there's nothing to be sorry about,' I pleaded with her, worried by the dry, deep noise coming from her lungs. 'I'm the one who's sorry that you're coughing – come on, too much courtesy can harm your health, you know that, don't you? I bet you even apologise to a chair when you bump into it.'

'Well yes, I do,' she admitted. 'And also when people bump into *me*. I guess you're right. My daughter's been wanting me to go to self-assertion classes, but I've never found the courage to go. Thank goodness she knows how to assert herself. It's too late for me to start on it now.'

'It's not, you know.' She was working against herself, I thought; she had to be shocked out of her civilised resignation, otherwise she wouldn't find the strength and the drive to recover. 'Listen, if you want to get well, you've got to claim your space and assert yourself. Stop apologising for being alive, will you please?'

'Is that what I am doing?' She smiled, wagged her head, pondered. 'Perhaps it is. Let's talk about it later, but only if you want to – you've got enough problems without bothering about mine. Oh, here I go again . . . See you at the lecture.'

I watched her moving slowly along the path – she was so slight, so easy to blow away – and I felt uneasy. But then I glanced at my watch and rushed back to the brown couch in my room. The non-stop train of the therapy tolerated no long halts.

The maid who brought me the castor oil, all too soon after the first red juice and the second enema of the day, handed it to me with a broad grin that clearly signalled rather-you-than-me. I shuddered, which made her grin even more. The colourless, viscous oil sat in a small paper container next to a cup of black coffee which was supposed to chase the oil through the stomach. It was the only coffee patients were allowed to drink and, perhaps to put off the caffeine cravers, it was ghastly – lukewarm and very sweet, just the thing not to get hooked on.

All right. Cheers. I knocked back the oil and gulped down the coffee. Horrible stuff, both. I had not swallowed castor oil since the age of ten or so, but when I had taken it, under maternal duress, it had always come thickly masked with fruit-flavoured syrup. Today, I suspected, the sickly syrup would make things worse. As I later discovered, the castor oil routine, hitting us every other day, provided a basic rhythm for life at the clinic. Castor oil days were bad days when nothing adventurous, such as a very short walk, could be attempted, and even attending a lecture had its hazards. They were bad days because the oil put us entirely at the mercy of our guts; one old lady even claimed to be dehumanised by the experience. There were times when I agreed with her. At other times I felt that we were making more fuss over taking two tablespoons of castor oil than Socrates had done over a full cup of hemlock. On the other hand Socrates did not have to take hemlock every other day.

When I entered the lecture room with my cassette recorder, I found Carl, still wearing his cherry-red jockey cap, talking to a dark-haired young woman. 'Come and meet Sarah,' he hailed me. 'Sarah can speak Spanish, she'll help us to communicate with the staff if the sign language fails.' I sat down beside Sarah. She came from New Mexico and looked markedly Spanish except for her light-green eyes, and she had come to the clinic with her mother who was gravely ill with leukaemia. She was too ill to get up even and I was asked to come to visit and give her some brief distraction. Did I think the therapy was good and would work? Well, yes, I said, I certainly thought so, otherwise I would not be there myself. Sarah nodded vigorously. She seemed out of her depth yet full of trust and hope, being both worried daughter and competent mother of three small boys, and as she talked about her family, she conveyed an extraordinary quality of love and courage. 'If my mother gets well,' she said, 'I'll set up a small Gerson information centre in our town. We've got plenty of people there who're sick with cancer.'

The lecture room was filling up. Becky fluttered in and sat down next to me. So many new faces were closing in, peering and talking and – mostly – flashing messages of tension or stress, that it was enough to give one people-poisoning or a bout of mettle fatigue. There were some individuals there whom I disliked on sight: an ugly, grumpy, middle-aged couple in absurdly youthful leisure clothes that made them look like overgrown toddlers, and a thin, manic, red-haired woman whose face resembled the imitation shrunken heads sold in some American souvenir shops. Togetherness, I decided, would have to be strictly rationed.

That morning's lecturer was Dr Hesse, the clinic's medical administrator, a tall, bearded man, overweight but light on his feet. His subject was the healing reaction or flare-up which, as we all knew from Jaquie Davison's book, could be very nasty. That morning he was going to give us the medical slant on what it was and how we were to deal with it. Dr Hesse looked us over, waited while two maids distributed the eleven o'clock liver juice, waited a little longer for our cassette recorders to be readied, and then began to speak.

'The Gerson programme is not necessarily for everyone,' he said, 'although medically the programme would cure the patient. Some are simply not willing to make the sacrifices and the changes in their life patterns that this programme demands. It's a very difficult, rigid and complex programme. You are being asked to take charge of your medical care. When you leave La Gloria, you'll be on your own. In fact, in most cases you'll be without an understanding local doctor to guide and care for you.'

A slight hiss arose from the audience, a hiss of regret

and dismay. Thank God for Dr Montague, I thought. May he not change his mind about looking after me.

'You are now in charge of your health,' Dr Hesse went on, looking at us very seriously. 'You must combine a very complete understanding of the programme with a great deal of dedication, will power and family support. A strong religious experience, trust and faith in God can also play an important role. So priorities must be defined and accomplished. And if these ingredients are not part of your make-up, it would be better if you were not to embark on what we consider an epic enterprise. It is truly epic, as you have in your grasp the means to regain your health.'

Becky and I exchanged a glance of shared apprehension but also of a semi-humorous, that's-a-fine-time-to-tell-us complicity. Yet beyond the apprehension I liked what I heard. Surely, turning the patient from passive object into active participant was the best way to mobilise his will and inner reserves. Also, invoking the patient's dedication, faith and trust seemed to round out the purely physical therapy into a more holistic one. What with Cos lettuce, originally from the island of Cos, and Hippocrates Soup on its daily menu, could La Gloria turn out to be the modern equivalent of the Greek healing sanctuaries I had been longing for?

Dr Hesse was now explaining the mechanics of the flare-up which, he emphasised, was the body's vigorous effort to detoxify and heal itself. The list of flare-up symptoms sounded appalling. Aches and pains, headaches, weakness, dizziness, cold sores, fever blisters, a coated tongue and weight loss of up to six or eight pounds were all possible. We could also expect intestinal spasms, great irritability, or else lethargy and discouragement. The tumour site might become painful and inflamed. Old scars and incisions might turn red, arthritic joints grow more inflamed. Former users of Valium, Librium, LSD and other drugs had to be prepared for even worse episodes, because as the old drug deposits were flushed into the bloodstream, they produced the same effects as they had done when first taken.

'Oh Gawd,' a man in the audience groaned, 'is it really worth it?'

Dr Hesse gave a half-smile, as if saying, 'I know how you feel,' and then went on at a measured pace. The main thing, he stressed, was not to panic when all hell broke loose during a flare-up, not to throw in the sponge and agree to be rushed to hospital or treated at home by conventional means. The body knew what it was doing, its self-cleansing and healing were not to be interrupted. Given the right conditions, which is what the therapy was all about, the body would do its job impeccably.

We all sat very still while Dr Hesse explained the correct handling of those healing crises. It was highly technical stuff and I vaguely wondered whether anyone in the throes of a major flare-up would even remember what to do, let alone do it. The cassette recorders hummed away in unison. A few people kept checking their machines while taking notes as well, which was surely the ultimate in anxiety. 'The remedies,' Sarah whispered during a brief pause, 'seem as bad as the symptoms!' Well, yes – thin gruel strained into the juices, large amounts of peppermint tea and enemas every two hours sounded highly resistible. And on top of all the physical torment we were even supposed to welcome flare-ups, the worse the merrier, and feel delighted if we ran a fever, because that meant that the immune system was not irreversibly damaged and that the body was beginning to reactivate its defences.

I tried to imagine how Mr Lennox would react to all this, but failed.

By the time the lecture was drawing to a close, most of us looked weary and chastened. I felt as if Dr Hesse had put us through a powerful mincer in order to break down whatever misconceptions we might have had

161

about the severity of our situation. If anyone had thought that having cancer and going on the Gerson therapy was a simple and easy matter, now was the moment to think again.

After the lecture, clutching our freshly delivered green juices, we drifted out onto the sunny terrace that ran the whole length of the upper building. Carl, who had had a few flare-ups, told us all he knew about the process, but, just like Dr Elsa, he could not forecast when those dreaded yet vital reactions were likely to start – the very thing Becky and I were longing to know. In theory, he told us, flare-ups should begin between the third and sixth day of the therapy, but often nothing happened for several weeks. And the first few reactions could be really foul, lasting for three days or more; later on they became milder and shorter.

'Personally I think,' Carl added, 'that the type of flare-up you get depends partly on your previous diet.'

'What do you mean?' Sarah asked.

'I'm not sure about this, but I think that the more junk you've been eating before going on the therapy, the faster you flare. Give your body a little bit of decent organic food and it'll start throwing out the garbage at once. There was a young guy here, a visitor who didn't go anywhere near the therapy. All he did was to eat the regulation Gerson food and drink two carrot juices a day. But within three days he went into a tremendous flare-up and was real sick for two days. He told us afterwards that he normally lived on large steaks, French fries and doughnuts.'

'What, no fruit, no salads?' Becky asked.

'Why, no . . . he lives in Alaska and fruit and vegetables are scarce up there. Still, I guess his flare-up made him think twice about his eating habits.'

'My Mom's got almost all the symptoms Dr Hesse has talked about,' Sarah said. 'Since yesterday morning she hasn't been eating or drinking, either. I was pretty scared at first, but she's probably flaring and then it's okay. I hope that's what it is – we've only got a week here.'

'Can't you stay a little longer?' Becky asked.

'No, we can't afford it. Ours is a big family, I've ten brothers and sisters and things are hard – we can only manage one week for my Mom. I'd better go back and see how she's doing.'

Becky and I accompanied Sarah to the lower building. Her mother, a sweet-faced little woman, lay in bed with an air of patient resignation. She looked very ill. Her eyes acknowledged us but she did not speak. Later I learned that she only understood Spanish. The room was chock-a-block with luggage, parcels, thermos flasks, trays of fruit, jars and papers, but above the chaos, on the chest of drawers, the plaster statuettes of the Madonna and Christ struck a note of divine order and hope. Clearly, Sarah and her mother were living the strong religious experience recommended by Dr Hesse.

After a brief while we walked on. There was not much territory to cover; all we could do was to tour the grounds and then return to the hilltop where Becky was staying. The upper block was much smarter than the lower one, with bigger, more pleasantly furnished rooms and specks of synthetic gold glittering from the textured paint on the ceilings. Walking along the wide corridor, I caught glimpses of patients resting, reading or chatting in their uncurtained rooms. The most striking person was an old, yellow-skinned man with blazing dark eyes sitting up in bed, surrounded by a bevy of sallow women in black; a sallow, dark-eyed youth sitting outside the room looked like a young version of the old man. They were Armenians, Becky whispered before retreating to her room; they stuck together, did not talk to anyone, did not take their meals in the dining room and seemed determined not to let the old man die. 'Poor old chap,' I whispered back, 'has anyone asked him whether he wants to live or die?' Becky smiled, shrugged and went into her room.

I needed a rest badly. There had been no idle moments since seven in the morning. At this rate I would have to rely on the enema breaks to guarantee me some peace, quiet and privacy, at least as long as I was up and about. Judging by Dr Hesse's lecture I could be felled by a flare-up any moment, and then (the child in me rejoiced) they would *have* to leave me in peace . . . after all, was this a clinic or an endurance course?

Outside the cottage I almost collided with a tall, handsome woman who came striding up the path at speed. She was middle-aged but her skin was like that of a young girl, and she had startlingly clear blue eyes with the kind of pure, snowy whites one normally sees in small children. 'Oh, hallo, I'm Charlotte Gerson,' she said. 'What's your name? Are these letters for you by any chance?' I could not believe my eyes. The letters she was holding up were all from England and all addressed to me, yet I had only arrived the previous day. 'So it *is* you – good,' Charlotte said as I introduced myself. 'Welcome to La Gloria. I'm glad you've managed to come . . . you sounded rather doubtful on the telephone. Look, I've got to rush now but I'll come and see you around two o'clock, okay?'

So that was Charlotte Gerson. After such a brief meeting the only thing I could consciously register was the facial likeness between her and her daughter Margaret; but what I could sense at an instinctive level was a powerful quality about her, a blend of energy and courage. I felt that she would be the right person to stand next to on an old-fashioned barricade, which was my symbolic yardstick, going back to the revolutionary fantasies of my adolescence, for classifying people. In those fantasies barricades were battlegrounds from which to attack tyrannies, so you had to choose your allies carefully. Charlotte, I thought, would know exactly what to do on a barricade; and there would be plenty of opportunities to decide whether my instinctive feelings were accurate or not.

But now the letters she had given me were burning a hole in my hand. I simply had to open them at once, and as I read them, greedily and with joy, I realised with a great leap of my heart that half a dozen friends had written those letters several days before my departure from London so that they should reach me soon after my arrival. So much thoughtfulness put a lump in my throat. For a brief while I felt re-attached to my world, no longer out of context.

That was the moment when I became dependent on friends' letters for my well-being. Throughout my two months in Mexico, mail from home acted as my happiness drug, my oxygen flask, my consolation and soul-warmer. To bypass the slowness of the Mexican post, all our mail went to an address in Southern California and was brought across daily by the clinic's driver who then took back our letters to the nearest American post office to mail. But sometimes he had no time to pick up the incoming mail or there were no letters for me, and whenever that happened I was overwhelmed by a childishly intense sense of disappointment and I would go back to my room and sulk under a pall of loneliness. Those occasions made me realise that my elemental 'inner child' was lurking much closer to the surface than I had thought, and that it possessed a boundless capacity for grief just an inch or two beneath my shell of apparent maturity and resilience – apparent being the key word. Still, at that moment, reading those precious letters, I had no inkling of my forthcoming troubles with my awkward and inconsolable inner child.

As soon as Charlotte arrived in my room after lunch, she wanted to know why I wore a bandage on my right leg. Surgeon's instructions, I replied, unwrapping my leg as carefully as if it had been an Egyptian mummy. Charlotte looked at my pathetic butchered leg and sniffed with exasperation. 'Poor you,' she said. 'And now, despite all this . . . magnificent surgery you have a secondary tumour in your groin. Stop wearing the bandage. Your leg needs air to heal properly. Just take great care not to knock your skin graft. Let's recap your case history, shall we?'

After I had answered her questions, I began to ask some myself and, with Charlotte's permission, recorded our conversation. 'If I get well, I want to write about my experiences,' I explained, 'so I'd better start collecting my material.'

Charlotte looked doubtful. 'Sure, you're welcome to do that, but it's too soon for you to start thinking about work. You'll probably have a lousy time before you start improving. Right now you should concentrate on the therapy. Come on, you only arrived yesterday!'

Ah, but yesterday was a long time ago, and I knew my needs and limitations and my regrettably low boredom threshold. So I switched on the cassette recorder and asked the question that bothered me most: was the excessive length of the therapy really necessary, or did the clinic insist on it to be on the safe side?

'Excessive? What's excessive about eighteen months or two years? It's nothing compared to the twenty or thirty years during which the body becomes gradually poisoned!' She had a fiery way of speaking which made an interesting contrast with her cool, fair-haired looks; she might have been a modern version of some invincible Valkyrie. 'The fact is that people today need longer to respond to the therapy than they did in my father's time, simply because they're more toxic. In the past thirty years the whole world has become more poisoned and polluted, so it takes longer and needs more hard work to heal and restore patients. We have to run faster and faster just to stay in the same spot.'

Yes, I conceded, I could see that, and was it not rather discouraging? No, not at all, she replied, because of the wonderful results they got despite the additional

166

difficulties. People were getting well, and there were among them some desperately ill patients who recovered on their own, without coming to the clinic, just by following the instructions in the book. There had been several people like that, not just Jaquie Davison.

'Let me tell you about Earl Taylor,' Charlotte said. 'Earl lives in Illinois. Fifteen years ago when there was no Gerson clinic and no doctor trained in the therapy, Earl was sent home from hospital to die. He was seventy, his prostate cancer had spread to his bones and the doctors said they were sorry, there was nothing more they could do for him, he should put his affairs in order.' At this stage in the story Charlotte made an expressive gesture which, I later discovered, was her signal to say that orthodox medicine had once again run into a blind alley; it was a fast yet dainty dismissive gesture, a spiralling, downward sweep of both hands as if the person represented by the hands had been trying to shake off dirty water or some other unpleasant matter. It was a gesture that said, in brief, 'Don't call us and we shan't call you, either.'

Earl, I gathered, was a widower of limited education who lived on his own. But through some health magazine he acquired Dr Gerson's book – and then found that it was way beyond him. So he telephoned Charlotte's sister who advised him to stick to the practical instructions and ignore the rest. He did just that and got well, and was now in his eighty-fifth year.

'And something interesting happened four months ago,' Charlotte added. 'Earl was doing some job in his house and he fell and broke a rib. When he went to the hospital because of the pain, the doctors assumed that his bone cancer had recurred and caused a pathological fracture. To make sure they gave him a whole bone scan, and they found no trace of cancer; he'd simply broken a rib. And he remains alive and well.'

Yes, I agreed, that was marvellous. And I liked the

way the clinic was abuzz with confidence and high expectations. But, but . . . 'Let's be realistic – what about the failures?' I asked, feeling almost rude to strike such a negative note, for there was something in Charlotte's essence that discouraged the contemplation of defeat. 'Surely you have failures, too?'

'Of course we have failures. Almost all the patients we get have metastasized cancers, like yours, which can no longer be influenced by orthodox methods. We get terminal patients who have somewhere between two weeks and four months to live. Some are in such terrible shape that they arrive on stretchers. A few months ago two patients died on the trip down here; we never even saw them. That gives you some idea of what we are up against. Beyond a certain stage the patient's organism is too far gone and can't be restored even with this therapy.'

'And what else can go wrong? Among patients who aren't too far gone? Surely there are failures among non-terminal cases, too?'

'Oh, yes.' She frowned. 'A lot of people don't follow the therapy properly when they go home from here. They find it too hard, too much work, maybe too expensive in some cases, or else the family isn't supportive and the patient eventually gives up. The fact is that we have a very high drop-out rate caused by practical problems; the therapy is not at fault, people could recover if everything could be handled properly for them. But some people feel that it's altogether too much trouble and they'd rather die than go through with it. And those we can't help.'

'Perhaps their motivation isn't strong enough,' I mused, 'or they can't tackle some underlying non-physical problem. What about the psychological or spiritual dimension of healing? Do you give patients any support in that area? I'm interested in that for professional reasons.'

Charlotte shook her head. 'The psychological side is

168

overrated,' she said flatly. 'All this talk about cancer being caused by stress is nonsense. Stress doesn't cause disease, but it may be a precipitating factor if the body is toxic and not functioning well. Stress may be the last straw, but it isn't the basic cause. Look here,' she said with a hint of passion, 'no one in this world leads a stress-free life, yet not everyone falls sick with some chronic degenerative disease. Why not? Because a healthy body is able to handle stress.'

'I see.' I swallowed hard. 'Does that mean that you don't believe in the cancer-prone personality, either?'

'No, I don't. Not the way it's normally presented. What I believe is this. When a cancer is diagnosed, it's been developing for a long time, during which the body has become toxic and depleted and its systems have broken down. Of course, in that condition the central nervous system is badly affected, the brain reacts, you become negative, miserable, depressed, emotionally upset. But all that is the consequence of the body's condition, not its cause!'

I could not accept that interpretation of the body-psyche link. It was too one-sided, too narrow to accommodate the endlessly subtle interactions of inner and outer, physical and intangible. But I was there to learn, not to argue. Besides, since my years of inner work and psychological exploration had not protected my body from the total breakdown commonly known as cancer, I felt it best to keep my objections to myself. I only asked Charlotte whether she saw no need to complement the therapy with counselling or other kinds of psychological support.

'No need at all,' she replied. 'If I wanted to oversimplify things, I'd say that once the patient's liver is restored, he can deal with his psychological or spiritual problems.' She rose and went to the door. 'I must go. We'll have other opportunities to talk, but just now try to settle in and learn the routine. That's the most important thing you've got to do.'

'Yes, I will. Isn't it a pity,' I added on an impulse, 'that you didn't become a doctor?'

'Good God, no,' Charlotte said merrily, 'I would have lost my licence long ago. As it is, I can do my work freely. I wouldn't have it otherwise.' And she was gone.

But some of her energy had stayed behind. I felt invigorated and boosted by our meeting. Charlotte had the true healer's ability to fill one with confidence and a fighting spirit. I could tell by now that she was a tremendous fighter herself and certainly barricade-worthy. Her dismissal of the psychosomatic aspect was a pity because it meant that La Gloria could not be a truly holistic healing centre on the Greek model. But then one could not have everything and, if I wanted it, I would have to supply the missing dimension myself; create and internalise the Asklepion of my fantasies. Since I normally felt more at home with the psyche than with the body, this would not be too difficult.

The rest of the afternoon was a patchwork of visits, juices, enemas, and a quick call from one of the physicians, Dr Arturo, whose Inca Indian features were even more impressive than those of the briefly glimpsed Dr Vic. I also survived the cataclysmic effect of the castor oil and managed to snatch twenty minutes' rest between two lots of knocks on my door. I understood the need for those constant intrusions and interruptions but I began to resent them. And as my irritation gathered strength, I suddenly came face to face with an astounding fact.

I had not smoked for more than a day; for thirty-three hours, to be exact.

What is more, until that moment I had not even been aware of such a major break in my habitual addiction. Yet in the past, on the many occasions when I had tried to stop smoking, after only eight hours' abstinence I used to paw the ground and twitch with irritability, unable to sit still or concentrate for more than three minutes. What on earth was going on?

The very thought of smoking promptly set off a mild craving and, of course, I had no cigarettes. This, in turn, pushed me back into the old conditioned reflex of my entire adult life, the panicky feeling that unless I could get hold of a cigarette at once, I would go to pieces in a spectacular fashion. At the same time I knew that smoking was the number one Gerson taboo and that patients caught smoking – or drinking, which I did not miss at all – were promptly shipped home. My contrasting urges, the wild desire to smoke and the fear of expulsion, swirled around disconcertingly in my mind, so I decided to take a walk and sort myself out. I noticed that there had been no craving or withdrawal panic until a few moments ago when I had begun to think about smoking, but by now all my cells seemed to shriek for tobacco and I rushed out without analysing the link between thought and craving.

To the left of the lower building there was a small grove with a Japanese bridge and a tame deer grazing in an enclosure. As I walked towards it, I saw an elderly man, a patient's husband, smoking a cigarette among the trees. Ah, here's my chance, I thought, with the low cunning of the addict. If I ask this man, he will surely offer me a cigarette which I could smoke later, in some safe spot, just this once before stopping for good. Yes, just one single smoke; after that I would not even want one. By now even the roots of my hair seemed to be twisting and clamouring for a soothing, solacing dose of nicotine.

I walked towards the old man, composing myself into a pattern of simple friendliness. Poor old boy, looking so lonely and miserable, he would probably welcome the chance to chat for a while and then offer me a cigarette. For all I knew, he was the only smoker on the premises; all the luckier for me to find him at large, with no one else in sight.

I was only a few feet away from him when a small breeze suddenly picked up his smoke and blew it straight into my face. Ugh. It smelt dreadful. A heavy, nasty, dirty, scratchy smell, off-putting, sickening almost. My clamouring cells and hair roots fell silent with shock.

I walked past the man in a daze and proceeded into the grove. My puzzlement was total. For some reason the cigarette smoke that had been the essential accompaniment of my waking hours for so many years had become offensive; what I had thought was craving was no more than a mental delusion which did not involve my body. I was having no withdrawal symptoms except for feeling that I ought to have them. I could not believe my luck.

I turned round and walked back again. Sniffed in reverse, the old man's smoke smelt just as awful. I returned to my room, feeling elated and mystified. I decided that if thirty-three hours on the therapy had cured me of a lifelong addiction – for there was nothing else to account for such a dramatic change in my reaction to cigarette smoke – then eighteen months on it should cure me of almost anything.

10

A POSSIBLE EXPLANATION of why I no longer wanted to smoke came a few days later, in one of Charlotte's regular talks to patients in which she combined solid information with encouragement. On that occasion she claimed that behind most addictions there was a deficient diet lacking in essential nutrients; once that was corrected, for instance by switching to the Gerson diet, the craving quickly diminished or ceased altogether. She quoted the example of a chain-smoking cancer patient who had delayed her arrival at the clinic as long as possible, convinced that she would be unable to survive without cigarettes; and yet within days of arriving she had kicked the habit without a pang. Just like me, I thought. If Charlotte is right and other smokers' experience also bears out her claim, then all the doctors, psychotherapists, hypnotists, heroic self-help groups and makers of anti-smoking preparations are barking up the wrong tree, and likewise all the hooked smokers, struggling to break free, are failing for the wrong reasons. Had anyone run a large scale controlled experiment, I asked Charlotte after her talk, to put the dietary hypothesis to the test? Not to her knowledge, she said with a shrug. No one would fund research into nutritional therapy because there was no big money in using sound, whole, unprocessed food as a therapeutic tool. 'Who wants to know about a method that would only benefit organic farmers and greengrocers?' she asked.

I registered a note of bitterness in her voice, a note

that recurred every time she talked about the steely resistance of the American medical establishment to alternative therapies, and to the Gerson therapy in particular. Sometimes her bitterness turned into downright anger when she discussed the vested interests behind the gigantic American cancer industry with its high turnover and even higher profits – an estimated twenty thousand million dollars were spent in the US on conventional cancer treatments every year. 'But, you see, the Gerson programme doesn't involve surgery, radiation or chemotherapy,' she would point out. 'Its use would cause massive unemployment among specialists, technicians, manufacturers and everyone else working in the industry. On top of that our results would make the immensely expensive official research programmes look rather silly. So we must be kept out of the way.'

And also out of California where, under State law, it is a criminal offence to treat cancer with anything other than the orthodox trinity, scornfully described as 'slash, burn, poison' by militants of the alternative camp. Yet California, with its mild climate and constant supply of organic produce, would have been an ideal location. To salvage the situation, the Gerson clinic and some other unorthodox cancer centres had been set up in and around Tijuana, close to Californian amenities but safe – and legal – on Mexican soil.

Even so, Charlotte told us, the American authorities launched regular attacks on non-toxic cancer therapies, dismissing them as quackery. 'But in my book,' she added with a flash of anger, 'quackery means that somebody sells you some expensive cure that he knows is going to fail – cures like chemotherapy, radiation and surgery. You only have to look at the cancer mortality figures to see just who are the quacks.'

In those early days at the clinic I sometimes wondered whether Charlotte did not exaggerate the medical establishment's obtuseness and hostility towards her late father's work. As I later discovered, she did not. But, on the whole, I had very little spare capacity to think of anything else than the demands of the daily round. Almost without noticing, I had slipped into the dawn-to-night Gerson routine and become body-centred to the exclusion of almost all else, not so much following the therapy as being run by it. Juices, enemas, doctors' visits, medication, injections, lectures, castor oil, meals, exercise, discussions with Charlotte, talks with fellow patients, reading and studying – every minute of the day was accounted for, every minute angled towards the aim of getting better. I just about managed to make time for the important job of letter-writing, of keeping in touch with my world. Without a typewriter I could only write short multi-purpose letters, asking the recipients to share my news with mutual friends. My growing commitment to the therapy was the quiet adult version of the zeal with which I had embraced noble causes in adolescence, and since I was surrounded by fellow sufferers operating on similar levels of commitment, I found nothing unusual in my total dedication to the treatment.

Also, I was now a member of a sub-culture which I found fairly familiar from my experience of the alternative medicine field in Britain; yet of course it was different, too. It was more specialised and more relevant, since what was at stake this time was survival and not, as it had been in London, the treatment of colds or the respective merits of acupuncture and zone therapy. Just being at La Gloria identified you as a member or associate of a sub-culture, because to have got there in the first place you must have been reading certain obscure health magazines or Church newsletters, known certain fringe therapists or listened to assistants in health food shops, or attended natural health conventions where Charlotte happened to lecture. Or, if none of that applied, people got to the clinic via the kind of personal grapevine that I had used. The only patients who came to La Gloria without any prior knowledge of the alternative world had been directed there by hospital nurses, after conventional treatment had failed to help them. Some nurses, with their ample experience of what orthodox cancer treatments did to patients, often advised advanced cases to try alternative therapies. At least nurses were free to do so, unlike those American doctors who had themselves recovered on the Gerson therapy but were forbidden by law or by unofficial pressures to prescribe it for their patients.

Belonging to the Gerson sub-culture made me feel somewhat like an early Christian might have felt, being a member of a small underground movement, cut off from the mainstream and, indeed, swimming against it, risking all, standing alone unsupported but convinced of an essential central truth that the majority did not see. But, unlike the early Christians, I and my fellow conspirators pursued a totally body-centred, practical and rational creed that promised immediate reward or punishment in this world.

Despite my dedication I had little to report during the daily visits of Dr Arturo or Dr Rodgers who took turns in making the rounds. I was still tired, but no longer with the deadly, pathological exhaustion of my last dark weeks in London. Tiredness apart, I was feeling moderately well and was no longer losing weight. My face looked less yellow, my eyes less clouded. When a puzzling scarlet mark appeared on my cheek, Dr Rodgers welcomed it as a healthy though tiny inflammation, and he was even more pleased when the bottom half of my sadly numb skin graft also turned red. Yes, great, but I wanted something more dramatic, a clear sign to show that my body was receiving the message. Why, for instance, did the lump in my groin not shrink or disappear? That question bothered me considerably. Out of sheer worry I must have sent the wrong thoughts to the lump, because within days it became more prominent and even harder. I no longer had to search for it with my fingertips, it was rising out of my groin like a miniature hill, having grown from its original almond size to a hefty walnut. It terrified me to watch that painless, rock-hard lump pushing up underneath the unbroken skin, like a sinister messenger from the depths. I panicked, but the doctors dismissed my stark fears. They assured me that the tumour was simply rising to the surface but not getting bigger, well, at least not in any significant fashion. Nor was I producing further tumours in the classical melanoma manner, so there was nothing to worry about. With considerable difficulty I took their word for it.

What I most wanted was a flare-up with all the trimmings, and that is what I did not get. Sarah's mother was still bedridden with hers and so ill that the family agreed to keep her at the clinic for another week, whatever that meant to the budget; Becky had started on her first healing reaction; up-and-about patients suddenly went missing from the dining-room, which meant that they were doing their duty and having flare-ups; only I was lagging behind. What was wrong with me, why did I not flare? Were my organs beyond repair, could they no longer respond? The waves of depression that were beginning to hit me had a familiar flavour. After some reflection I understood that I was reliving the bewilderment and depressions of my childhood when, as an only child untrained in the tribal laws of proper families, I had often found myself the odd child out among my peers, out of step, guilty of some unwitting trespass. What had I done now, why was I not flaring like everyone else?

At last, on my tenth day at La Gloria, I woke up feeling very queer: dizzy, leaden with fatigue, my skull brimful of cotton wool and insecurely attached to my neck, my stomach distressed. Alberta found my temperature above normal and showed me the thermometer with a beaming smile. I beamed back. My mouth tasted of blotting paper soaked in contaminated cider,

177

but I felt pleased, longing for my body to put up a really good – which meant really bad – show. When I staggered out of the cottage and saw Carl strolling along the path, I called out to tell him that I was feeling utterly dreadful.

'That's great! You look dreadful, too – I'm very glad,' he said, giving the correct Gerson response that would have sounded unkind in any other setting. 'Seems like you'll have your flare-up at last. Go to bed, the maids will bring you all your juices and meals.'

'I don't want anything,' I croaked happily before returning to bed. My head was aching, and I felt slightly seasick but nevertheless pleased as I dozed between the juices which I somehow managed to drink. But by mid-afternoon, instead of sinking into the multiple distress sketched out by Dr Hesse, I suddenly recovered and felt quite normal – and accordingly disappointed. It had been a false flare-up, my body was not responding to the therapy, it was too late, I might just as well go home and die.

'Stuff and nonsense,' said Carl when I told him about my doubts. 'Absolute nonsense, Bee. You and I are going to get well, I know it, so quit complaining.' He sounded as if he had just received from heaven a confidential guarantee of our recovery. 'You may not have a proper flare-up for weeks – so what? You've got nearly two years to play around with. What's the hurry?'

All right. No hurry. I felt sheepish, though no longer desperate. I turned my attention instead to the literature of the alternative field. The clinic had no library, but some patients were glad to pass round their own books which were of common sub-cultural interest, and I decided to read them all. The first one I borrowed was *Confessions of a Medical Heretic*, by an eminent American physician, Dr Robert Mendelsohn. It amounted to a zestful, thorough and total condemnation of modern medicine as it is practised in the US. 'I believe that modern medicine's treatments for disease are seldom effective, and that they're often more dangerous than the diseases they're designed to treat,' the highly qualified Dr Mendelsohn states in his introductory chapter, and at La Gloria, where most patients bore the marks of unsuccessful orthodox cancer medicine, his uncompromising views made him into an instant cult hero.

I was particularly struck by a sentence in his chapter on *Ritual Mutilations*, which is his term for misguided or unnecessary surgery; a chilling though slapdash sentence which curtly states, 'Modern cancer surgery someday will be regarded with the same kind of horror that we now regard the use of leeches in George Washington's time. It was shown to be irrational thirty-five years ago.' By weird coincidence I was reading that very sentence on my terrace when I looked up and saw a tall, sad-faced man walk past me. From the lopsided shape of his thin jacket I could see that he had lost to surgery not only his left arm but his left shoulder as well, and that, judging by his grey face and very presence at La Gloria, the radical amputation had not solved his problem. I watched him with great fellow-feeling, wanting to find out more about his case, but he vanished as quietly as he had appeared and I never saw him again.

There were other, less tragic short-stay guests whom we committed patients watched with scorn. These were the well-heeled Americans who found the premises too modest, the rules too strict, the diet too Spartan, and who departed after a day or two, scattering indignation in their wake. One of them, a glamorous middle-aged woman journalist from New York, cross-examined me at length about the therapy, only to conclude that despite the bad prognosis for her spreading cancer she could not possibly undertake the Gerson programme. She listed several reasons in support of her decision before coming out with the final clinching factor. 'This therapy,' she declared, 'would disrupt my lifestyle.'

'So would death,' I suggested with more honesty than tact.

She scowled, snorted, rushed back to her room and left La Gloria the same day.

I went on reading every book and magazine I could borrow until I was able to compile for my own use an outline of Dr Gerson's personality and character. From my sketchy sources he came across as a strong, gentle, quiet man, absorbed in his work, absent-minded enough to wreck four bicycles in minor accidents and to fall down a coal chute. Above all he was modest, unpretentious and tenacious. Without exceptional staying power he might have packed up medicine altogether or suffered a breakdown in his prime, for his whole life was punctuated by tragic reverses and disappointments. It was as if Fate had offered him marvellous opportunities with one hand, only to snatch them back with the other just before fruition. Yet even with such a cruel stop-go pattern Dr Gerson had achieved unique results; what might he have done on a smoother track?

Two episodes of his career stood out as particularly bitter milestones. In 1932, when he was fifty-one, he was granted full facilities at a Berlin hospital to prove that his dietary treatment could cure even hopeless cases of tuberculosis. After long and painstaking efforts he was due to demonstrate his results before the Berlin Medical Association, in a presentation that, he knew, would make his therapy widely accepted and open the door to further pioneering work. But five weeks before the scheduled demonstration Hitler came to power and Dr Gerson left Germany with his wife and three daughters. (Many of his relations who refused to follow his example perished in Nazi concentration camps.)

Another dazzling opportunity came – and went – in 1946 when Dr Gerson, by then resettled and working in New York, was allowed to present five of his recovered cancer patients to a US Congressional committee, the first physician to be able to do so. What was at stake was a Senate Bill that, if passed, would have provided funds for research into his therapy. The presentation was an unqualified success, but the lobby supporting conventional cancer therapies defeated the Bill by four votes. And that was that. The solitary immigrant doctor with his German-flavoured English and remarkable results was once more left out in the cold, partly ignored, partly persecuted by various medical organisations, including the American Cancer Society, which listed his therapy under the heading of 'Frauds and Fables'. But he went on working, alone, amid increasing difficulties, and died at the age of seventy-eight, in 1959. As the final irony of his strange fate, the New York Academy of Science invited Dr Gerson to become a member – two months after his death.

Only once did his life pattern seem to have worked in reverse when, instead of reducing a great chance to ashes, it turned a severe handicap into a tool of discovery. As a young man Dr Gerson suffered from long, incapacitating bouts of migraine which his medical colleagues could not cure. So he began to experiment with various diets and soon found that a saltless regime of raw or freshly cooked vegetables and fruits, especially apples, banished his migraines. He recommended the same diet to his migraine-stricken patients, with excellent results. Soon one of those patients reported that his severe attacks of migraine had ceased – and his *Lupus vulgaris* (skin tuberculosis) was also healing. Since *Lupus* was considered incurable, Dr Gerson could hardly believe the man's claim – or the evidence of his own eyes. But there could be no doubt. The *Lupus* lesions were healing. And he was forced to conclude that the diet was not so much healing a specific illness as restoring the body's own ability to heal itself – of migraine, *Lupus*, TB, or whatever was wrong with it. That was how his revolutionary work began, leading, in due course, to his startling success with terminal cancer cases.

It was melancholy to ponder the ups and downs and might-have-beens of Max Gerson's career nearly twenty-two years after his death, in that small, modest Mexican hospital that was the only tangible token of his life's work. I felt sure, and so did other patients, that if in 1946 the Congressional committee had voted funds to conduct research into Gerson's methods, the therapy would have been streamlined and simplified long ago, allowing patients to follow it without having to retreat from normal life for nearly two years. But that was all speculation and theory. In practice we had to get on with the job and not grumble.

I did grumble, though. The food was beginning to irritate me, especially the boiled onion smothered with raisins that revolted me whenever it appeared on the menu. I had consciously switched off my normal appetite for enjoyable meals, but my instinctual side refused to obey and I began to have vivid dreams about forbidden foods. I was in the same position as St Antony being tormented by inadmissible tempting visions in the desert; but while his visions had been of fat and randy naked ladies soaring through the air, in my gastronomic desert I dreamt about eating exquisite salty, savoury and cheesy dishes or snacks, always in a French setting. One dream took me back to a certain *boulangerie* off the Rue Soufflot in Paris which sold feather-light puff pastry twists with luscious creamy cheese fillings; another one deposited me in a rustic restaurant in the Auvergne where spicy grilled sausages were served with lashings of pale, golden matchstick *pommes frites*. The odd thing about these highly realistic dreams was that in each one I was able to take and eat what I wanted, without having to pay for it. It was a neat piece of wishful thinking about breaking the diet without ill effects. But if that was what my unconscious was tempting me to do, it remained unsuccessful, and suddenly the dreams ceased.

182

But I still grumbled: about the monotonous Hippocrates soup, the out-of-order telephone which stopped me from ringing Hudie, which I very much wanted, or getting a call from him, the inefficiency of Marcos Aurelios who officiously wrote down my needs and requests every morning and then disappeared for the rest of the day without producing the goods. Nothing seemed to be right. One morning, when I was in vigorous mid-grumble, Sarah took me by the arm. 'Come on,' she said, 'you need a change – let's go and look at the sea at Rosarito. Luis the cook is willing to drive us there, and if we leave now, we'll be back in time for your liver juice at eleven.' I jumped at the chance of getting out of the place and within minutes we were off, streaking along the impressive highway that ran past La Gloria.

What I saw from the car was less impressive. The scenery was heartbreakingly ugly. Barren, dusty earth, universal dirt and mess, a chaotic mixture of abandoned cars, pylons, shacks, sheds, rashes of puny vegetation, unfinished concrete structures, a string of yellow tractors, large notices advertising PRECAUTION, brash signs offering building sites FOR SALE. There were scruffy motels advertising LUNCH DINNING and one even serving BAREAKFEST. Several shops along the road were selling MUEBLAS ESTUFAS which, I presumed, meant upholstered or maybe stuffed furniture, and near Rosarito we passed souvenir shops of varying awfulness. People were burning acrid-smelling rubbish all over the place and everywhere there were beautiful children, scampering about in small bands or herded by women shaped for, or by, continuous pregnancies.

At last we reached the humble, scruffy seaside town of Rosarito and stopped by a deserted beach. I got out of the car and hurried along the sandy strip, leaving Sarah and Luis behind. After the onslaught of ugliness and poverty along the road, the crested blue rollers of the Pacific were so magnificent and beautiful, such a majestic counter-argument to my petty despair, that I had to experience their impact on my own. Also, I would have found it hard to explain why I was crying. I was not sure myself, but I suspected that the sea was confronting me with the ultimate in connectedness and oneness that made my own isolation terribly painful. At any rate I wept briefly and bitterly, straight into the whipping wind, feeling homesick, lonely and infinitely crushable; then I blew my nose and returned to the car.

'You must be feeling stronger, otherwise you wouldn't grumble,' Becky suggested later that day when I visited her and, contrary to my original intention, gave her a brief list of my discontents. Becky was in bed, suffering from a strong flare-up, but her elegant spirit and humour shone through her obvious malaise. 'The honeymoon with the clinic is over, don't you think?' she went on. 'The therapy makes you feel better, so you start noticing the flaws and drawbacks.'

'You may be right,' I said. 'There's a lot of inefficiency here and I do wish the staff spoke some English; I find this state of non-communication trying. But I'm also more irritable than usual, don't know why. Does carrot juice lower one's flashpoint? It should do the opposite, surely?'

'Wait until you get a flare-up,' Becky said. 'You'll find it makes you marvellously forgiving and tolerant.'

She looked pale and exhausted after two days of splitting headaches and nausea, but recovered in time for Charlotte's Saturday afternoon lecture, which was the week's highlight at La Gloria. This time her lecture was attended not only by patients, their helpers and visitors but also by a coachload of American hospital sisters and administrators who were touring the unorthodox cancer centres of the Tijuana region as part of a 'continuing education programme'. I watched them file into the lecture room. Almost all of them were overweight, quite a few were obese and shapeless, waddling in the manner of the very fat whose legs no longer meet. They were living testimonials to a truly dreadful diet. If health professionals look like this, I thought, God help their charges.

Charlotte began her talk with a brief summary of the therapy and then homed in on her main theme, which was that as the treatment is non-specific, in due course it enables the body to heal all its troubles, not only its most threatening disease. 'The body is not selective,' she said, 'it won't heal one or two of its problems and neglect the rest. Sometimes we are surprised to see how even some very old and tricky health problems disappear with this kind of total healing. For example, we had an eighty-year-old lady here, with very high blood pressure and chronic bronchial catarrh. Both cleared up on the therapy. Then she wrote to us from home to say that she'd regained her hearing, and that her cataracts had disappeared. We didn't even know about her cataracts, she hadn't bothered to mention them, but they cleared up all the same. That's what we mean by healing.'

She launched into further examples, giving the names, addresses, ages and exact case histories of former patients who were happy to serve as living testimonials to the therapy. Eric Goodman, for instance, who once had cancer of the jaw, plus severe heart fibrillation, migraine, sinus trouble, arthritis, haemorrhoids, insomnia and lack of energy. 'He went on the therapy because he didn't want to have his jaw removed,' Charlotte explained, 'which was all his doctor had to offer. Not only did his cancer heal, he also lost all his other problems. He'd been given six months to live and that was five and a half years ago.'

A murmur ran through the audience. Some of the hospital sisters exchanged astonished glances and tiny nods, signalling interest and satisfaction. They grew even more impressed when Charlotte presented the case of Melva Blackburn who had been suffering since 1940 from kidney disease, gradually adding to it heart and coronary artery disease, an enlarged liver, a whip-lash that refused to heal, diabetes, pneumonia at least twice a year, osteo-arthritis all over her body, obesity, fatigue, confusion and premature senility.

This time the hospital group tittered with incredulous amazement. My own reaction was that anyone who lived on despite so many serious complaints must have had a fabulous constitution – or an exceptional zest for life.

'Melva started the therapy in October 1979,' Charlotte went on, 'fifteen months ago, and now she's fine – off all drugs, including insulin, which she started taking in 1965, fifteen years ago. It's an interesting time scale; fifteen months of therapy achieving what fifteen years of orthodox treatment could not do. Last fall she went back to her physician. He was astounded to see her in such good health – and then he wanted to put her back on drugs!' Charlotte's voice had risen to an indignant near-shout and her eyes were bright with anger. I could imagine her confronting a massed band of orthodox doctors and demolishing their arguments with cold facts and hot anger. I could also see how she would put up the backs of vaguely sympathetic but unconvinced medics who might expect softer arguments. But then I realised that Charlotte was La Pasionaria of the alterna-tive medicine movement, with a unique role to play; the patient, gentle persuasion would have to be done by someone else.

Then she switched over from past case histories to the presentation of current patients on the mend, sum-moning to the rostrum some of us who were sitting unsuspectingly in the auditorium. The first one to be called was Bert Brehaut, a cheerful young man who was recovering from the destructive side effects of drugs prescribed by his doctors over twelve years. His was the familiar story of taking one drug that soon necessi-tated the use of another and so on, until the patient almost disappeared under the cumulative reaction of harsh chemicals with unpronounceable names. All Bert had wanted in the first place was pain relief for an injury. What he got instead was partial pain relief – and a tangle of drug-caused problems, including powerful food allergies that eventually reduced him to eating nothing but potatoes. By the time he came to La Gloria, accompanying his wife Marie who had cancer, Bert was suffering from constant pain, prostatitis, arthritis, multiple allergies and severe liver damage. When he realised the extent of his problems, he stayed on and started the therapy together with his wife.

'I've been able to cut out all drugs,' Bert told us, 'and the pain is going. I can eat all the food we get here without ill effects and I can sleep normally, lying in bed instead of sitting up as I used to do, because of the pain. It's great to function properly again,' he concluded with a shy grin. Charlotte patted him on the shoulder. We applauded vigorously.

Next came Bert's wife Marie, a thin, pale girl with tousled hair and a bizarre story. Since a mastectomy two and a half years before, she had felt ill, weak and generally unwell, but her doctors accused her of cancer psychosis and dismissed her symptoms.

'That's typical,' Charlotte interjected. 'They try to blame the patient for their failure to heal.'

Marie nodded. 'I kept going back for check-ups,' she went on, 'but the tests showed nothing wrong. Five months ago, after a special check-up for insurance purposes, I was told that I had no trace of cancer. But I had such awful pain in my sternum,' she said, touching her breastbone gingerly, as if expecting it to break, 'that at last the hospital did a bone scan and they found that I had cancer of the sternum and ribs and also right into my lungs. The doctors told me that I had two months to live. That was two months ago.' She smiled but her voice trailed off; she had run out of steam. Gently, Charlotte helped her off the platform and finished her story for us.

'Marie came here in severe pain,' she explained. 'We took her off drugs and she obtained pain reduction through coffee enemas, but it took her three or four days to get rid of all the pain; and then she promptly started painful healing reactions. She's been through a really rough time. But,' Charlotte raised her voice to a triumphant pitch, 'despite all that she's already put on eleven pounds, she can breathe freely and sleep soundly and her condition is improving all round. Please note – she's still very ill. But she's begun to recover from metastasized cancer which is officially incurable.'

This time the applause was even louder and longer. Much of it came from the hospital group whose members must have seen many patients in Marie's condition rush downhill towards certain death. There was something stirring and compelling about the interaction between Charlotte and the patients on the one side, and the audience on the other. We were being shown a balanced mixture of the strictly factual – for all patients had fully documented medical histories – and the near miraculous – for contrary to the official prognoses they had recovered or were improving. Personally, I found the testimonials of the still struggling, far from cured patients even more exciting than the success stories of the long-healed former patients who were the heroes and heroines of the Gerson gallery. The difference between the two groups was the same as that between the Church Militant and the Church Triumphant, or between muddy privates and golden generals who had won their wars. I realised that the analogy with the Church was out of place, for the supernatural had neither room nor role in the therapy and we were not asked to accept or believe anything without suitable proof; it was simply that my Catholic background was breaking through into my spontaneously chosen metaphors, as it had done when I had compared the clinic's patients to early Christians in a flimsy catacomb. And

188

also at that moment when I, too, was a muddy private, with a growing tumour in my groin and total uncertainty about the future, I found that my feelings were tinged with something resembling religious zeal. They contained growing commitment, trust, faith in the therapy, a willingness to move mountains or, at least, to have a good try.

Charlotte produced two more patients, both improving but far from healed. One young woman, suffering from an inoperable brain tumour, told us that she was getting fewer and fewer seizures, could see well and had no mental or muscular disturbances. She was as bright as a new penny, poised and purposeful. The other patient, a beautiful blonde woman, had been heavily drugged by her doctors since childhood for a grand mixture of complaints, until she suffered a severe breakdown and had to live in a darkened room in a state of severe depression. 'It took eleven weeks just to wean her off drugs,' Charlotte explained. 'We often find that cancer patients are easier to get into good shape than overdrugged ones who don't suffer from malignancy. That gives you some idea of the destructive effects of drugs.' The ethereal blonde smiled, nodded and left the rostrum. She looked as frail as the finest eggshell porcelain, but was clearly anxious to test her growing resilience. This time the applause was gentle, as if we had feared that a loud noise might crack her.

The doors swung open and three maids appeared, bearing glasses of tomato-red juices on large trays. Charlotte took one, too. 'What's that stuff?' one of the hospital ladies wanted to know.

'Raw liver and carrot juice,' she replied, and laughed when a collective shudder seized the hospital group. 'No, it's not like that at all, it tastes quite nice.'

'Why do you drink it? Are you sick?' another hospital lady asked aggressively. I grinned. Charlotte looked almost indecently fit and un-sick.

'I drink it because I want to remain well,' she said.

'Some of my father's oldest patients who are in their eighties and even nineties are still active and working, with good eyesight and good hearing, because they've been following certain rules over the years. I'm doing the same – investing in a healthy future. That's why I drink quite a few juices.'

'All right then, what are those rules one should follow?' one of the fattest visitors demanded.

'Keep your liver functioning, your potassium level high, your food healthy, and you'll remain fit,' Charlotte replied. The meeting was over.

I switched off my cassette recorder and watched the departing hospital group with a strong awareness of them and us; us including everyone at the clinic, even the patients I liked least. Charlotte's lecture had filled me with a lively if temporary sense of community with everyone on the therapy. 'This tape,' I said to Becky, 'and all the others I'm recording here will be very precious back in London. I'll play them for comfort when I feel rotten, or against loneliness when there's no one to understand what I'm going through.'

We strolled out into the grounds, deep in thought. 'I can't help feeling,' said Becky in her soft, slightly apologetic voice, 'that this therapy is a kind of benevolent medical time bomb. It's all there, ticking away quietly, it could blow a whole lot of current medical practice sky high and change our whole approach to health and illness, but very few people know of its existence and no one knows how to set it off.'

'If my dearest friend Catherine were here,' I mused, 'she'd simply ask us what *we* are going to do about that. I suspect it's people like us who'll have to set off the bomb, because no one else will do it. That's one more reason for us to get well, isn't it?'

'Yes, absolutely.' Becky nodded with unaccustomed vigour. 'And then we can celebrate together. In London! I'll come over with my husband and meet you and your man, and we'll have a slap-up meal – '

'Of salad and Hippocrates soup and jacket potato,' I cut in, 'and gallons of fresh carrot juice. I'll be able to supply you with endless juices, I'll have all the equipment on the premises!'

We hugged each other and laughed, exhilarated by the thought of a joint celebration at the end of a long, dark journey. 'At a pinch,' I said, 'I might be able to put you up for a few days unless your husband is very large – you see, I live in a tiny house.' We went on planning and joking in high spirits, relishing our fantasy of liberation, when I suddenly felt an icy chill in the pit of my stomach and I knew with dreadful certainty that Becky and I would not celebrate our joint recovery in London or anywhere else. The only thing I did not know was which of us would fail to survive. But a moment later the chill vanished and I dismissed that glimpse of doom with a shrug. *Che sera, sera,* I thought. Besides, my brown couch was waiting.

11

THE SENSE OF community inspired by Charlotte's talk and presentation of patients stayed with me for a while and I found myself getting more and more involved with the people of the clinic. We all had a story to tell, and once we started sharing and swapping the kind of rough basic experiences that had brought us to La Gloria, relationships automatically formed. Sharing the same disease in most cases, and the same therapy in all, was a strong link, even if we had very little else in common. Besides, contact with each other was our only distraction apart from reading. The lectures on various aspects of the therapy were repeated every week, so that after attending one series there was nothing left to learn. Only Charlotte's Saturday talks were always on a different subject. There was no television on the premises for health reasons, since the radiation which is emitted is considered harmful. And there was no other entertainment within easy reach – none, some pessimists claimed, this side of Los Angeles, hundreds of miles away. So we had to rely on each other for contact and conversation.

Some of these contacts brought more anxiety than joy. Emily, the pretty old lady with the malignant rash on her face, sometimes broke off her lively chatter and declared that in the silence of the night she could feel the cancer eating away her flesh like a real crab. Nonsense, we all shouted whenever she said that, what a silly thing to say. But besides making a lot of noise, like frightened primitives trying to chase off devils, we watched her anxiously, wondering whether she was in fact getting worse.

I found these occasions harrowing, for I had grown fond of Emily, but my worst, most despondent moments were caused by Mike, the gloomy Dane. Since our joint arrival at La Gloria he had grown even more gaunt and colourless and he walked around with his right hand permanently resting on his waist which made his elbow stick out at an awkward angle. I thought he looked like an unhappy stork nursing a broken wing. If you asked how he was, he shook his head with a thin-lipped quarter smile and explained that it was a fast-growing lump in his armpit that stopped him from letting his arm hang loose and straight.

I suspected that Mike derived some satisfaction from not getting better. At any rate he cast a thick shadow. We all dropped our voices and toned down our laughter when he appeared. The way he ignored us – never starting or contributing to a conversation, never taking an interest in anybody's problems or ideas – suggested total coldness and rejection; he even seemed to reject and belittle the therapy on which our survival depended. Mike's universal negativity depressed me so much that sometimes I found myself wishing that he had been suffering from some other cancer, not melanoma, for I was uneasy about having anything in common with him – and then I felt guilty for harbouring such mean thoughts about a fellow sufferer.

But there were others to compensate for uncongenial or alarming company. Guy, for instance, a likeable young man who was crippled with MS (multiple sclerosis). When he first arrived at La Gloria, he could hardly walk even with the aid of two sticks and a supporting arm on either side. He also kept losing his balance: once, in the dining-room, three of us could just about stop him from crashing headlong to the floor. But after eleven days on the therapy, four of them spent in a violent flare-up with raging temperatures, Guy was able to walk unaided, almost normally, carrying a stick but not leaning on it. 'Hey, look at me,' he yelled as some of us cheered him on. 'My left leg's been useless for seven months. You can see how my shoe's worn right down on one side where I had to drag my leg along – and now it's functioning again!' We could not have been more impressed if he had started walking on the bright blue water of the swimming-pool. Yet deep down I felt sure that had he done so, Charlotte would have ordered him to stop at once, since the chlorinated pool was strictly out of bounds and walking on water would have been no excuse for breaking the rules.

Later that day I sat on the terrace with Guy and his sweet-and-sour, wisecracking wife Barbara, talking about his experience. 'Oh yes, I know that in MS you can get temporary remissions,' Guy said quietly, 'I've had one or two myself. But I can tell that this isn't just a remission. It goes much deeper, somehow. It feels completely different.' Both he and Barbara were visibly stunned by his sudden improvement. They looked both young and old, vulnerable and battle-toughened, contemplating this latest twist in Guy's saga of self-inflicted sickness that had begun with dope-taking at the age of fourteen, leading to two serious liver diseases at sixteen, unrecognised MS at twenty-one, heavy medication of the wrong kind, and eventually a diagnosis of fast deteriorating MS and total despair. Now he was in a good strong lifeboat. Whether he would stay in it was another matter. By his own admission he lacked self-discipline and was afraid that he might relapse into drug-taking and chain-smoking. But for the moment he was fine, and through the peculiar alchemy of La Gloria which allowed us to participate in each other's moods, Guy's startling improvement boosted our collective confidence by several degrees.

Personally I needed a boost badly. My tumour was still growing, and the doctors' reassurances did not convince me entirely. In fact, for a day or two I was deeply scared. The lump should have shrunk or at least remained unchanged; I could find no excuse, no rational explanation for its increasing size. If I had not been at La Gloria, in the very middle of the battlefield, eternally busy with the therapy, I would have got into a very bad state. As it was, at that moment, exactly two weeks after my arrival, my body produced two encouraging changes. The painful arthritic knots on my right index and middle fingers that had troubled me for years became terribly sore for a day – and then stopped hurting altogether. I could squeeze the top joints as hard as I liked without feeling any pain. Moreover, the knots were shrinking. This pleased me enormously. I knew that arthritis normally grew worse, not better, with the passing of time, but since mine was doing the opposite, I could assume that Dr Gerson's claims about the total nature of the healing were correct, and that, therefore, the therapy was bound to work against my cancer, too (it was just plain unfortunate that my body's healing priorities were different from mine). For another thing, I was glad to shed a bad genetic legacy. Twenty years before, my mother had developed arthritis in those same two fingers and they had then quickly become deformed. The crippling process had only stopped after she had reluctantly, and without faith, attended a spiritual healing service. The deformity, however, had remained. How odd, I thought, contemplating my fingers, that both my mother and I should develop arthritis in the same spot and then, odder still, that we should both arrest the process by two different kinds of unorthodox treatment. Who could tell which of the two, spiritual healing or carrot juice, was the more unusual?

The other encouraging sign was that when the results of a new set of blood and urine tests arrived, I found that I was free of diabetes. 'I told you so,' Dr Elsa said casually when I gave her the good news. 'You didn't believe me when I said that your diabetes would go without specific treatment, but now you have proof. Look, on this therapy even severe diabetics can normally come off insulin after a month, so it's not surprising that your mild diabetes has cleared up in two weeks. I hope you believe me now?' I did, with pleasure and gratitude. The therapy had freed me from a second genetically inherited complaint, for my mother was also a diabetic.

The following morning Sarah left for home with her small, silent mother who did not seem to have improved after her long flare-up. She should have stayed under constant medical supervision, but the family funds had finally run out and Sarah had to take her back to New Mexico. I was sorry to see them depart with their mountain of luggage crowned by a brand-new juicer which was to be the backbone of further treatment at home. I realised what an important role Sarah had played among us with her unsinkable cheerfulness which brightened and often defused our heavy moments. She also radiated trust, and in a place where most of us were seriously ill while the attendant relatives were seriously worried, Sarah's uncomplicated faith in a benevolent (and strictly Roman Catholic) deity who ensured the general rightness of things, acted as a refreshing drink of spring water. And now she was leaving. A few of us stood outside the administrative block to see her off. 'We'll miss you,' Becky called out. The rest of us nodded vigorously. Sarah tried to reply, but the car drove off and there was nothing we could do except wave and wave until it disappeared in the traffic.

A few days later Sarah wrote to me to announce the death of her mother. 'The therapy came too late for her,' she had written. 'But at least she died peacefully at home, surrounded and loved by the whole family. I am so glad we didn't let the doctors do any more dreadful things to her at the hospital. It was God's will.'

After some small ups this was a big down. The news saddened me, not just for Sarah's sake but also because I found it hard to accept that the therapy had failed to save a patient who had done all the right things. My disturbed reaction to the death of that almost unknown old lady made me realise how much faith I myself had invested in the Gerson programme; faith and the unconditional belief that the therapy always worked. But that was dangerous nonsense. Charlotte would have been the first to denounce it. Besides, leukaemia patients normally came to La Gloria after receiving massive doses of chemotherapy that had destroyed the last shreds of their natural defences without curing the disease, so their chances were slender. Yes, I knew all that and gradually I got things back into perspective. But on another level something non-rational in me had to go on believing that as long as you stuck to the rules and kept your psyche in reasonable order, you were bound to get well. If something had destroyed my faith at that stage, I think I would have returned home to die.

As I had still no sign of a flare-up and wanted to save money, I asked Dr Rodgers whether I might move to La Mesa clinic, La Gloria's sister establishment a few miles away. La Mesa was for patients who, like me, were in a stable condition and did not need constant medical care. The diet, the provision of juices, injections and medication were the same as at La Gloria, but there were no lectures or demonstrations, the doctors did not call daily and Charlotte visited only once a week. In return the charges were lower.

'Sure, you may move to La Mesa next week,' Dr Rodgers agreed. He was a jolly man, bearing a vague resemblance to Clark Gable. 'There's just one condition. If you go into a heavy flare-up or produce some other problem, you must come back to La Gloria at once. I'll go on seeing you at La Mesa anyway.'

That sounded fine. Feeling restless, I arranged to

move at the end of my third week at La Gloria. Without a flare-up I was beginning to find the slow, steady rhythm of the Gerson treatment hard to take. Heavens above, nothing was *happening*. Well, nothing much, at any rate, since losing my diabetes and watching my arthritis heal could not be dismissed as nothing. Only these developments, which anywhere else would have been sensational, did not seem to be quite enough at La Gloria where you quickly acquired high expectations. For that reason I did not stop to ponder how much better I was feeling every day, or that my colour had changed from a sickly grey-yellow hue to a much clearer, nearly rosy shade; those changes I simply took for granted. The trouble was that I had not yet become attuned to the quiet pace of natural healing. All my former experience of disease and cure had been dramatic. The removal of my tonsils at ten and of my appendix at nineteen had been major upheavals, as had my cancer operation, but in between those brusque interventions I had experienced long, normal, doctorless spells of well-being. Now, however, I was seriously ill yet there was no drama, no drastic action, no grand spectacle or breathless emergency, and I knew that short of dying I would not produce any upheaval for a long time; but despite that I could not abandon my monotonous cure and live a normal life. That was a strange formula that weighed heavily on my impatient nature. Moving to La Mesa would at least make a change. Apart from Carl and Becky there was no one I would miss from La Gloria, and Becky was to go home soon while Carl was planning to move to La Mesa himself.

In the midst of that restless patch I had a dream that pulled me up sharply, as if a deep, kindly warning note had been sounded behind the cacophony of my fractured state of mind. In the dream I saw myself sitting at a square table with two robed Masters who were teaching me some important knowledge. Then a third one, the Master of Personal Space joined us. The curious thing was that I could only see the back views of our foursome.

It was the kind of numinous dream that is best saluted with respect before any interpretation is attempted. The unseen faces of the majestic Masters indicated that the dream was reporting about an inner process that was going on far below – or far above – the level of normal consciousness. The square table was a symbol of earthly wholeness; it could also signify stability, the four elements, the body and tangible reality. In my current situation the two latter meanings seemed most relevant. All right, so while outwardly I was fully occupied with the non-stop demands of the therapy, performing the day-long dance of the thirteen juices and five enemas, deep inside I was learning something important about the long-neglected earthly-physical aspects of my life. Who were the two unidentified teachers? I did not know. Only the latecomer, the third Master, had a clear identity: Personal Space – and I did not have any just then. All that relentless body-stuff had invaded my personal space, my inner space, the lot. Perhaps I should start working on that at once. Perhaps.

The dream and its haunting afterglow made me realise how few of my dreams I was able to remember now. The constant exchange between waking consciousness and unconscious material brought up (or down?) by dreams, which had been a useful and often entertaining routine of my pre-therapy life, had slowed down to the point of near extinction. I also realised that I was not meditating any more at all, not even to the extent of taking quick maintenance doses of stillness and recollection. That was strange, unusual, certainly bad under the circumstances; perhaps the main drift of the dream was to warn me that my inner life was badly slipping. But if it had been that, would the Masters had sat with me at the table? I tried to work this one out, but the constant interruptions – by maids bearing fruit platters, juices, jugs of fresh coffee or piles of towels – made me give up in desperation. I decided to start meditating again as soon as I was resettled at La Mesa.

Shortly before my move Charlotte came to ask whether I would like to meet Karen, a new arrival from London who was in a serious condition. 'She's only twenty-one,' Charlotte explained, 'she's on her own and a long way from home. You're the only other Londoner here – it would be nice if you kept an eye on her.' I agreed gladly and we went off at once to call on Karen.

Her appearance shocked me. She was a beautiful girl, with the delicate features of noble ladies in medieval miniatures, but her face looked as white as a sheet, with deep black shadows under her eyes; her arms and legs were like sticks and her abdomen was bloated with fluid that made her seem five months pregnant. Oh God, I thought with a pang of helpless pity, she will not last long and she hasn't lived yet. It seemed cruelly ironic that cancer had given her the same grotesque shape that African children get through starvation. Karen was obviously exhausted by her trip and very weak, but she rose to greet us and smiled and talked as if we had been meeting in a pleasant social setting. So much grace and courage somehow made the situation even sadder.

Karen was full of cancer, Charlotte told me afterwards. She had been ill for a year with severe pains in her knees, chest and stomach and had been treated with a variety of drugs, including steroids, until at last her doctors had diagnosed cancer of the breast, stomach and possibly of other organs, too, by which time no orthodox treatment had been possible. 'So she's here now,' Charlotte said briskly, yet with a shadow of resignation in her voice, 'and we'll do our very best to pull her through, but it's going to be tough. We're up against not only the cancer but also a load of poisonous drugs in her system, and as you know, that makes healing doubly difficult.'

Karen stayed on her feet for two days, eating her meals in the dining-room and making friends with everybody, before going down with dreadful bouts of sickness, pain and weakness. I visited her several times a day, wondering whether she was having a flare-up or a final flare-out of life. All I could do was to beg her to drink a little juice or a drop of soup, as if I had been coaxing a sick child to take a tiny mouthful for Daddy's or Teddy's sake, and she did try, but it was an obvious struggle to take in any nourishment. Other patients called, too. Karen's youth and touchingly good manners, that did not crack even under extreme stress, brought out everybody's protective instincts. Marcos Aurelios, that champion of inefficiency, took to sitting inside her door, keeping a devoted dog-eyed watch on her until she had to ask him to go. We all feared the worst.

But two days later, to my enormous relief, Karen arrived to visit me early in the morning. She still looked like a beautiful thin apparition, not quite of this world, but the black shadows under her eyes had gone, together with her dreadful pallor, and, most astoundingly, her stomach was no longer bloated. 'Look, it's flat again,' she said in her clear little voice, patting her front. 'It looks normal, doesn't it? I didn't think it would go down that quickly.' I trotted around her twice, inspecting her new silhouette and hardly daring to believe my eyes. The difference was extraordinary. 'Well, Karen,' I said, 'the only thing to say is "Phew!" and dance all over the grounds, but that'll have to wait a little longer. Do you know that Chinese saying: even the longest journey begins with one step? You've just taken that first step – congratulations! But don't forget that the trip has only just started.'

She nodded and smiled. 'Oh, I know. Because of all those drugs I was being given in London I'll have to be on the therapy for three years instead of two, to get really well. But . . . I've no choice.' She said it calmly and with great composure, as if mentioning a minor nuisance like losing a bus ticket or having to postpone a holiday.

'I admire your cool,' I told her. 'The good thing is that even if you have to do three years, you'll still only be twenty-four when you regain your freedom, and then you should be good for another seventy years or so!' Yes, she agreed, that was a worthwhile investment. Since I was to leave for La Mesa that day, I gave her my address and asked her to contact me when she got back to London. When or if, I wondered, seeing her back to her room.

I wondered about the same thing a little later, saying farewell to Becky. Goodbye and *au revoir* until London, keep in touch, keep up the therapy, next time we meet we will be big and strong, see you, see you. When or if. She wore her favourite kaftan in subtle shades of green, beige and brown, colours which she thought matched the salad, the Hippocrates soup and the coffee enemas of the therapy to perfection. I felt I was leaving an old and close friend, yet we had only met three weeks before. As if reading my thoughts, Becky lightly touched my hand and said with a lopsided smile, 'My mother believed that past the age of twenty-five no one could make really good new friendships – how wrong she was! Thanks for being such a good bad influence on me. I feel nicely subverted and you've saved me the bother of going to self-assertion classes. In future I'll just assert myself wherever I go and be really tough about it.'

Somehow I did not see that happening. The anxiety I felt for her had to be diffused and neutralised before her fine intuitive antennae had a chance to pick it up. So I deliberately broke up the slightly emotional under-tow of the moment and lowered it to a more down-to-earth level. 'Better practise some aggro while you're still

202

here,' I suggested. 'At home it'll be more difficult. And better start at once – do you realise that you'll be home in a week and that's only thirty-five enemas away? I'll have to get through at least two hundred before I can start packing . . . and then there'll be another few thousand enemas for both of us before we can give up the habit. It's not an elegant way to measure time, but I find it highly relevant just now.'

We laughed and embraced carefully – impulsive gestures are not for weak and underweight people – and then I got into the car, next to the impatient driver. A moment later we were swallowed up by the Tijuana-bound traffic. My stay at La Gloria was over.

12

AS BUILDINGS GO, La Mesa was pleasant enough – a modern two-storey block, built in the Spanish style around an oblong courtyard, with the windows facing inwards and an arcaded gallery linking the upstairs rooms. The trouble was that this well-groomed building stood in the middle of a dusty, litter-strewn settlement that lay between the roaring highway and a range of bare hills, so that the moment you stepped outside the clinic, you found yourself in a landscape of desolation. The other drawback was that, unlike La Gloria, this clinic had no garden. Apart from some flowering plants in pots and some hanging baskets, the sole greenery in sight was a plastic grass carpet in the courtyard.

I disliked the setting and the aridity of the place. Having got used to La Gloria, I now felt exiled once again, rootless and displaced. But my spirits rose when I was allocated a whole apartment with two bedrooms, a large sitting-room, a bathroom and a former kitchen turned into an enema parlour. 'Oh yes, it's great to be able to spread yourself,' said Doris, the dignified black ex-nurse whom I had met at La Gloria and was glad to find here. 'But let me warn you, the apartments are meant for two patients and if the intake shoots up, someone may be moved in with you.' Not if I can help it, I thought. My greatest, most burning need was for privacy.

When Maggie, the manageress, came to greet me, I was intrigued to discover that she was only twenty-one. Having heard about her efficiency and style, I had expected someone older and weightier than this slim, pretty, Mexican version of everybody's favourite kid sister. Maggie spoke fluent English. She also had the poise of a fashion model and an air of qualified optimism. When I asked her what it felt like to be responsible, at her age, for a whole clinic, she claimed it was terrifying – but said so with a broad grin that expressed the opposite. As I later discovered, in moments of crisis she could look frighteningly grave, like some ancient Inca angel of doom pondering the imminent collapse of the Universe; but then she would giggle and become her cheerful self again, rushing around in four-inch stiletto heels or driving the clinic's van as if she had been breaking in a bronco. Maggie had star quality. After a few minutes' conversation with her I felt reassured about my stay at La Mesa.

From now on, she said, I would have to do some therapy chores myself; easy ones, like refilling my medication box every night for the next day instead of having it delivered with my breakfast, taking my morning temperature and learning to inject myself with the daily dose of liver extract and vitamin B12. The nurse would show me how to do it, she would even go on injecting me if I found the needle-sticking routine awkward. 'But if you don't learn it now,' she warned, 'you'll need skilled help at home, too.' So that was why this was a halfway house: halfway between the total hospital care at La Gloria and the totally do-it-yourself future at home. I asked for a week's grace with the self-administered injections, which was granted. Maggie handed me containers full of my usual capsules and tablets and referred me to The Book for the correct dosages, should my memory need refreshing.

When I walked back to my room I almost bumped into Mike the Dane who was standing in the upstairs gallery, gazing at a potted begonia. 'Ah, you've got your daily rations,' he observed. 'At least the stuff won't do you any harm, even if it doesn't do much good.' He said he had arrived from La Gloria two days before; I thought he looked more ill and dejected than ever. 'Can't stand this place,' he muttered, 'and I'm getting weaker. The only person who's worse than me is the patient in Room 7 – make sure you visit her, she's got the worst melanoma I've ever seen.'

Blast you, I thought, as he returned to his room, keep your blackness to yourself, I have got enough trouble controlling my own. Even in those few moments he had once again made me tense and uncomfortable; it seemed to me that at some deep level he was egging on the destructive process in his body to do its worst and show the world that with melanoma you could not win. This poor man, I thought, needs exorcising; or I do, every time we meet.

Fortunately, as if by magic, the antidote appeared at once. I heard some strange noises and when I looked down into the courtyard, I saw two white-haired women, one tiny and elf-thin, the other pretty massive, waltzing around with gusto and singing an off-key version of *You must have been a beautiful baby*. They looked slightly manic and totally captivating. Downstairs, someone laughed. A woman called, 'But you're still beautiful, both of you!' Then I heard the thin wailing of an accordion. How lively, I thought; perhaps there is life after the third liver juice of the day.

I ambled downstairs and introduced myself to the dancing women who had by then collapsed onto a garden sofa. 'Oh good, a new face at last,' said Phyllis, the massive lady. 'This place isn't half as much fun as La Gloria, we need some fresh input to keep us going. That's why Lettie and I sometimes go off the rails and fool around a bit, to liven up the place. What's your problem? I have cancer from my throat to my . . . seat, if you'll pardon the expression, but I'm getting better. Well, I've been perking up ever since I passed a large tumour, you know, through the usual channels. Don't know where it came from but it's made a terrific difference,' she declared in her powerful fruity voice and then launched into a monologue about her grandchildren.

Compared to her bulk and cheerful loudness, the tiny woman, Laetitia, looked almost insubstantial and patrician. She was very old but she moved with great agility and had the serene – if shrivelled – face of an old-fashioned little girl, complete with enquiring child's eyes and an Alice-band in her straight, shoulder-length hair. 'My father was English,' she said on hearing that I came from London. 'Come and talk to me some time. I live in the corner room over there; I call it my cage. People may tell you that I'm mad – well, I'm not. And if they tell you that I'm eighty-seven, that's not true, either.'

I promised to visit her soon and returned to my quarters for a rest. The house Bible lay on the coffee-table. I opened it at random and to my amusement found myself reading this verse: '. . . and had suffered many things of many physicians, and had spent all that she had, and was nothing bettered, but rather grew worse.' Ah yes, the case of the woman with the twelve-year haemorrhage, poor soul, although judging by the description it might have been a modern American cancer patient in search of a cure (I had heard enough stories from patients to make the connection). I closed the Good Book and, just to amuse myself, opened it at random once more. This time I found myself gazing at the chapter in St Matthew that sounds like a faith healer's wish-fulfilment, with Jesus raising a dead girl, curing a man of the palsy and enabling a dumb man to speak, whilst being attacked by the Pharisees. How random is my random scanning of the Gospels? I wondered; is there some weird unconscious mechanism by which my mind, focussed on alternative medicine, directs my hand to open the Bible on stories of unorthodox healing? No, no, that was a bit fanciful. So I tried once more and got the same result, this time hitting on the case history of the man blind from birth who has his sight restored by Jesus. I remembered it well, but now, from the Gerson perspective, the story seemed to possess a fresh, weirdly amusing relevance, especially in the newly sighted man's exchanges with the Pharisees who cannot, will not accept the miracle worked by Jesus and react like a group of disapproving orthodox doctors grilling the healed patient of some fringe therapist.

What amused me most was how the Pharisees, after a lot of tut-tutting over the breaking of the Sabbath law (it is bad enough to work a miracle, but to do it on the Sabbath is unforgiveable) refuse to believe that the man had been blind in the first place. Well, well, I thought, nothing has changed; today's corresponding orthodox ploy is to say that the original diagnosis had been wrong and that the patient had never suffered from cancer or arthritis or whatever so-called incurable complaint the alternative therapist had healed. Poor born blind man: having been vilified by the Pharisees and cast out from the synagogue, he must have wondered whether being given sight had been such a good idea, after all.

At that moment another juice arrived. I put the Bible down and dismissed my triple find as an amusing coincidence.

Shortly afterwards the clinic's secretary turned up. 'We've received a letter from your surgeon in London,' she said, waving a sheet of paper. 'It's just arrived. Now we have your case history at last.' Of course, I had signed a form on arriving at La Gloria, authorising Mr Lennox to release all relevant information to Dr Hesse.

'Oh good,' I said. 'Let me see it, please. I know what's in it, anyway, except for the long words.' The girl handed me the letter and went off on her rounds.

Mr Lennox's message contained no great surprises until I reached the last paragraph where he described the discovery of the lump in my groin. 'When I reviewed her again on the 29th December,' I read, 'this lump was still present, and therefore I advised a block dissection of the groin.' Meaning, I now knew, the removal of all the lymph glands from the area.

My stomach performed a violent lurch. So all that talk about the need for a biopsy had been eyewash. He had known all along that the lump was a secondary tumour and the biopsy would have turned into radical surgery, even though he had not expected it to work. God, was I feeling sick – the shock of our last meeting hit me again, as if Mr Lennox's letter, impeccably typed on embossed paper, had filled the air with some dark threat, as if the man himself had been about to materialise and ask me to stop messing about and have my nice operation before it was too late. But this was nonsense, I thought, trying to steady my shaky insides; come now, calm down, all that is past history, you are safe, you are all right. Yes, quite. But I still needed a few deep breaths to coax myself back to normal.

I returned to the first paragraph which described the start of my illness. 'Histological examination showed that the lesion was an invasive malignant melanoma,' I read without surprise, but then a mighty inaudible ping sounded inside my head and I remembered how the man in the gospel story had to prove to the Pharisees that he had been blind until Jesus had healed him. The next thought followed logically: if I get well on this crazy therapy, things being what they are, I may have to prove that I did, indeed, have cancer, and the only indisputable proof of that happened to be in my hand. This was the moment to secure it.

'It's just a thought,' I said to the secretary when she returned, 'but when I get back to London, my physician will need my early case history. Will you please let me have a photocopy of this letter? I see no point in troubling the surgeon twice.' Oh sure, she said, quite right, no problem, leave it to me.

A few days later she brought me a photocopy of Mr

Lennox's letter. I put it at the bottom of my therapy information file and felt much better for knowing that it was there. Whatever the future was to bring, at least my past history was now secure.

My brief brush with the Bible might have been designed to prepare me for some of my encounters at La Mesa. During the next day I met several out-and-out Christian fundamentalists among the patients – people who prayed aloud before opening their mail or switching on the washing machine in the laundry room, people who hummed hymns and wore pins with JESUS FIRST in bright lettering, people who took every opportunity to proclaim their faith and hand it around, as if it had been a box of extra-special chocolates, for the unredeemed to help themselves, people who thought they knew all the answers although they had not even learnt to formulate the questions. I found their card-carrying public piety embarrassing, even irritating at times. The trouble was that despite their smug missionary zeal the people concerned were thoroughly likeable, warm and open characters, so that I could not simply put up my metaphorical shutters and pretend not to be there. All I could do was to avoid certain subjects and take care not to expose my flank to the honeyed darts of pop theology.

One of the reasons why I resented the fundamentalists' over-simplified, ruthlessly joyful faith was a kind of inverted envy. I certainly did not want what they had, but I longed with increasing anxiety for my own inner life to break out of its paralysis, stir, wake up and reconnect. Despite all efforts I was still unable to meditate or even recollect myself in stillness, and my favourite prayers had lost their meaning. What had once been limitless inner space was now a scary dark void which I could not cross. It felt as if an impenetrable steel door had slammed shut, cutting me off from my inner resources or even from my soul – whatever had become of my soul, I wondered stupidly without finding an answer. The feeling of inner alienation, which at first I had regarded as a temporary difficulty, caused by the shock of my illness and the stark demands of the therapy, had become a permanent state. My life had lost its innermost dimension; I was left with the outer structure, the scaffolding, the husk. And still my dreams remained elusive. All I knew was that I dreamt a great deal every night, but the dreams themselves, my customary keys to the changing climate and scenery of my unconscious, remained inaccessible. All this made me feel deprived and disorientated. It was tough enough to spend all day on a body-and-gut-centred routine; to be banished from other areas of life even at night was a severe punishment.

On top of it all, the sneaking discomfort in and around my left shoulder-blade was getting worse. It was not a pain or even an ache, just a sense of pressure and vague dislocation, but my constant awareness of the area signalled that something was wrong with it. On my third morning at La Mesa, I examined myself in the shower and to my horror found a lump under my arm: a painless but unmistakable lump, not matched by anything on the other side. Moreover it was a lump on my left side, which until that moment had been my good side as opposed to the damaged right. I turned off the tap and just stood there shivering, unable to move. Why hast thou forsaken me? something inside me asked. The shivering got worse. I wrapped myself in a bath towel and lay down on my bed. A lump in the armpit, I reckoned, was the beginning of the third and no doubt final act in this ghastly show I was involved in; from now on it would be downhill all the way, following Mike's example. What with no flare-up in nearly four weeks and now a fresh swelling in the armpit, the therapy had obviously not stopped the spread of the disease. It was not working for me as it was not working for Mike and, presumably, for other unknown melanoma patients struggling along at home.

211

For the first time my trust in the therapy was seriously faltering. I felt like a foolish creature who had tempted Fate, backed the wrong horse and would now pay the penalty. But then I thought of Charlotte with her blazing integrity and strong, no-nonsense attitude to the therapy. She was the last person to be naively optimistic or make unfounded claims, and she thought that I could be cured and was doing well. So. Well, then what was going on? I uncurled from the foetal position (so useful inside the womb, in moments of distress outside it, and also when taking an enema) and began a spell of full yoga breathing. Slowly my heartbeat returned to normal. Wait and see, wait and see. Dr Arturo's visit was due soon – better get dressed and gather my wits.

'No, it's not another tumour,' Dr Arturo concluded after a thorough examination. 'It's a swollen gland. Quite harmless. You may even get a few more in the next few weeks, but you mustn't panic if that happens. Don't make the mistake of so many cancer patients who think that every physical change is tied up with the cancer and invariably means something dreadful. It isn't so. That kind of fear can cause as much damage as the disease itself.' He looked at me thoughtfully with his dark Amerindian eyes; of all the doctors at the clinic he carried the greatest authority. 'Have you ever had any problem in or around your left armpit?'

I shook my head. And then, with a start, I remembered: in the past twenty years I had discovered a swollen gland roughly in the same spot at least two or three times; on each occasion I had immediately reported to my doctor or gynaecologist, expecting something nasty, only to be told that there was nothing to worry about, the lump would go, and would I please type my articles or scripts more slowly, irrespective of deadlines. Why had I forgotten all that, I asked Dr Arturo, feeling sheepish.

'It's quite natural to forget inconclusive episodes,' he

212

answered a trifle wearily. 'If this has been a recurring problem over the years, it may flare up quite strongly at this stage and then clear up for good. Like the arthritis in your fingers, or any old injury or problem that needs further healing. But you mustn't get scared when that happens. Panic is the worst thing for you, it upsets and disturbs your body's functioning.'

'Oh, I know that,' I said. 'You may find this hard to believe, but I used to give talks on the exact way in which emotions affect the body. But lumps terrify me. Lumps mean that I'm getting worse. You see, I don't feel all that secure now, I'm not convinced that I'm improving. So I keep my cool on an intellectual level, but it doesn't take much to throw me off balance.'

'I understand. But you've got to work on this.' He bent down and pointed at my right shin and towards the ankle where the skin graft was permanently red and angry-looking. 'That inflammation,' he said, 'means that the healing process has begun, the body is trying to repair that massive surgical damage. Let the body get on with the job and don't wonder why it's not doing something else instead.' He got up and went to the door. 'I assure you that if you were getting worse, you'd look and feel quite different. That's one of the drawbacks of this therapy – patients feel so well that they get restless and impatient and expect instant miracles. And those we can't produce. I'll see you again soon, unless it's Dr Rodger's turn next time.'

He was right, of course. I felt foolish and slightly ashamed of my terrified reaction to the lump. But my panic had also been useful. I now knew that it was not enough to follow the physical therapy. I would also have to monitor my moods and mental attitudes instead of simply drifting along with them, so that if something went wrong I had a firm base to stand on. What I really needed was someone to help me carry my load. I would have given anything for an hour with Catherine or John, but they were half a world away and there was no one at the clinic for me to talk to. Clearly, keeping my psyche straight had to be another do-it-yourself task. I promptly began to ease myself into a more confident and relaxed way of being and decided to brighten my days as well as I could – go for a walk every afternoon between the second and third liver juices, spend time with cheerful patients, get somehow to Tijuana for a hair-do, remain positive and optimistic come what may.

What did come the very same evening was an elderly couple from La Gloria, a raucous wife with her mute husband, and they were moved in with me to share the apartment. This blow surpassed my worst fears. I was suddenly corralled with two people instead of one, moreover with two people whom I had carefully avoided at La Gloria and whose behaviour now drove me to instant despair.

Anyone might have thought that Tom, the tall, slow, speechless old man with his uncomprehending eyes was the patient, attended by Lily, his strident wife, but no, it was the other way round, which only went to strengthen Lily's power base. Lily had quite a lot of cancer and she announced this as she announced everything else – in a loud, mocking, I-dare-you-to-contradict-me kind of voice. Tom, whose mind no longer worked, was not much trouble, except for his inability to distinguish between doors, so that he often barged into my bedroom or the enema parlour instead of going to the bathroom or leaving the apartment. But that was a small nuisance compared to the devastating effect of Lily, whose voice penetrated walls and ear-plugs, who walked about nearly naked which – at her age and in her condition – was a bad idea, and who somehow managed not to understand anything about the therapy, which inspired her to ask me the same silly questions over and over again.

My irritation rose by the hour. During the night I had to knock on the bedroom wall three times to silence

214

Lily's metallic monologues, but then she and Tom began a shuttle service to the bathroom, banging doors, running the water, flushing the lavatory endlessly. Never mind about staying positive and optimistic, I fumed inwardly, I cannot even get any sleep; this nuisance has to stop.

'But I have nowhere else to put them!' Maggie pleaded in the morning when I protested against her unfortunate billeting. 'We're full up! You were the last single patient occupying a double apartment, I had to put them in with you. I'm sorry, there's nothing I can do.'

'I'm sorry, too,' I said, 'but you've got to do something. Tell Dr Arturo that I'm being difficult or unreasonable or whatever you like, but I can't go on sharing with those people.'

Maggie looked unhappy. 'The telephone's out of order again,' she said, 'and even if I could ring Dr Arturo, he wouldn't be able to help, he's got nothing to do with accommodation. But listen,' she said, dropping her voice, 'this hasn't been announced officially yet, but we're going to move soon to a much nicer building by the seaside where everyone will have separate rooms . . . no one is happy about these shared apartments. So please be patient, we'll be moving soon.'

'Ah, well, that's different,' I said. 'How soon is soon?'

'A week, perhaps.' She sounded hesitant. 'And meanwhile if an apartment is vacated here, you'll have it at once. I promise.'

But no apartment fell vacant, the workmen preparing the new clinic ran into grave plumbing problems, and my enforced cohabitation with Tom and Lily continued. Things got worse every day. The old couple had taken over the sitting-room, so I stayed most of the time in my bedroom which was too hot during the day and had no table on which to write. Every afternoon I went up into the hills, not without difficulty, for the muscles in my right leg had seized up and hurt badly. But once I

215

had struggled uphill just high enough to get a wide view over the valley and beyond, I felt as if a tight band had fallen from my chest, letting my lungs expand again. The hills were poor and denuded after the failure of the rainy season, yet everwhere I saw blades of fragile grass and tiny plants of astounding beauty sprouting from the dusty soil. I was also much intrigued by some birds that I could hear but not see; their well-modulated call, sounding like a cheeky question, came from all directions, but all I could see of the birds was some fluttering movement close to the ground, half obscured by clumps of dry weeds.

I became attached to that humble, downtrodden spot. It made me feel free and secure, if only because there was no one else around and I could enjoy the endless expanse of the sky in privacy – the only privacy of my day. Just sitting on that hillside was enough to put things into perspective and give me some insights. Not all of them were enjoyable. It was up there, for instance, that I first realised how my life was being gradually stripped down by the therapy, or perhaps by a larger experience of which the therapy was only a part. I had already been stripped of my feminine vanity and its symbols, my scent and make-up; my tint was fading, letting the grey and white hair show through the remaining brown. It seemed a beastly irony for my hair to go salt-and-pepper at the precise time when salt and pepper were strictly banned from my food. My looks were being altered and eroded and I could not fight back.

More importantly I had been stripped of my professional life, my work, joys and pleasures and, above all, of the company of the people I loved. I felt dreadfully lonely, living among strangers when I so badly needed some meaningful human contact. But the nearest friend I could think of lived in Dallas, another three lived in New York, one in Australia, the rest in London; this was loneliness on a global scale. And as if that had

216

not been bad enough, I had also been stripped of my options, my inner life, my privacy; I had no guaranteed future, no plans or prospects; nothing, I concluded, except a wobbly sense of identity and a great, abiding love for a handful of people. Was that enough to survive on? Everything else was going, going, gone. Some of my cherished values and standards toppled and crashed even while I was examining them, like cheap crockery in a fairground booth. Control over my surroundings, a rigid code of conduct, a passion for perfection, for foolproof advance planning and defences against all possible snags, the latter impossible in itself – all these things, which added up to the structure of my days, had lost their meaning.

But there was even more to come. I had one more old, cherished value to lose, namely the almost foolproof self-control that had enabled me since the age of four to deny and repress my anger, staying in control at all times and only lashing out verbally, with deadly precision, when the provocation grew too strong. That apparently indestructible self-control gave out the same evening during dinner. I do not know why it happened at that moment. Admittedly the company in the dining-room was dismal: Mike and Tom gloomy and quiet as the grave, Lily making enough noise for three, Phyllis discussing tumours in unsavoury detail, and Laetitia arguing with two garrulous women about the best way to cook rice. Their voices grated, mingled and clashed until I knew that I could not take another minute of it without screaming or hurling the linseed oil at the chandelier. The vehemence of my irritation surprised me. I hurried out of the dining-room and walked up and down, up and down the length of the courtyard, trying to let off steam, choking and tense to the point of pain. My last coherent thought was that the idiotic conversation around the dinner table had nothing to do with how I felt. My sense of stormy disturbance and doom came from some other source which I could not identify.

A second later I was overwhelmed by anger of a kind I had never experienced before and therefore did not know how to handle. It felt dark, murderous and as unstoppable as a volcanic eruption; I thought that my skull and chest would split open and spatter everything with thick, black lava. I rushed upstairs and retreated to my bedroom. My heart was pounding. I could not breathe properly. I wondered whether I was succumbing to some mysterious psychosis, but then even that question became irrelevant, because my anger left no room for reasonable thoughts. I was powerless against that anger; it invaded and occupied me, like a powerful army overrunning a pathetically defenceless land, and I suddenly knew, or thought I knew, what it would feel like to attack and fight someone to the end. Who, me? Yes, me. Really me? It seemed so. I did not like that, it scared me, especially because there was no one to attack and fight or kill; my violent aggression and rage were unfocussed. The pressure within my skull grew stronger.

I pulled my pillows to the edge of the bed and started bashing them, holding my arm straight and bringing it down viciously from shoulder level, as in a judo breakfall. Pillow-bashing was a classical way to release pent-up anger. I had often suggested it in the course of counselling to inhibited clients, and now here I was, beating the stuffing out of the clinic's pillows – and feeling only slightly better for it. My anger needed something stronger to release it. I opened my bedroom door and slammed it shut as hard as I could, but it did not make a sufficiently loud noise, so I started pushing the furniture around, kicking and shoving like a mad-woman. I also swore under my breath fiercely but monotonously, for my small stock of bad words was insufficient and I had to repeat them again and again, which diminished their shock value. Throughout this

218

strange performance a very small part of me that had remained sane observed my actions, and although it could not stop me, at least it linked the raging major part of me to a reality that stood outside my fury. Even so, I still had a lot of destructive energy to channel, so I picked up the *Los Angeles Times* and began to tear its countless pages into long and narrow strips, scattering them all over the room. Strong brown paper would have made a better tearing sound, but I had to make do with soft newsprint. The front page contained an interview with a distinguished Californian cancer researcher (I paused in my dance of destruction to read the piece) who was quoted as saying 'Until now we had been approaching cancer from the standpoint of destroying it by surgery, radiation or chemotherapy. The exciting thing is we now have evidence we can approach cancer physiologically by enhancing natural processes.' Oh really, is that so, I raged – what else is new, you pompous fool, are you discovering in February 1981 what Dr Gerson knew fifty years ago? . . . but I cut out the article all the same for my press file and then continued to tear up the rest of the newspaper.

The sheer effort of turning some one hundred and forty pages into paper spaghetti calmed me down. Once more I felt like myself. I also felt bewildered by my experience of infantile rage, for that is what it had been: the murderous irrational aimless barbaric rage of a three-year-old child, acted out by an adult. You horrible brat, I said to myself. I felt exhausted and embarrassed and went to bed at once, not even trying to identify the raging toddler within.

That outburst was the beginning of a more or less continuous state of anger that lasted for ten days at varying levels of intensity. I was angry, snappy, irritable, impatient, jumpy, unkind, both hypersensitive and hypercritical, mean and aggressive. Part of me was aware of my dreadful behaviour and grieved over it, but the major part went on being nasty and destructive.

I tried to keep my venom to myself so as not to upset others, but did not always succeed; I tried to defuse my anger either in my bedroom or during my afternoon rambles, but some of it always stayed behind and blew up at awkward moments. Even letters from home did not help because I knew that, at least for the time being, I was not the person they had been written to. My mother, Hudie, Catherine and other friends would have hardly recognised me in the childishly horrid, angry person I had become. Much as I missed them, it was just as well that we were unable to meet.

What shamed me most was the pettiness of my anger and the way in which I resented weakness in others while being so blatantly weak myself (ah, straightforward projection, the small sane voice at the back of my head observed – hating your own faults in others). Yes, sure, shut up, the bully voice snapped back, projection or no projection, I do not care. I was particularly nasty to the squat, bovine nurse who administered my daily injections. She brought out the worst in me with her clumsiness and obvious stupidity, and I was rude to her although – or perhaps because – she spoke no English. I felt sure that the tone of my voice conveyed the message vividly. But then as soon as she left my room with her neat tray and bewildered face, I regretted my harshness and wanted to apologise.

On the ninth day of my season of rage my friend Carl arrived from La Gloria, looking as sane and sardonic as ever. Judging by the amount of luggage pouring out of the clinic's car, he had come to stay. I was delighted to see a familiar face and hurried downstairs to greet him in the courtyard. 'Thank goodness you're here,' I cried. 'I badly need someone to talk to and you'll do very nicely!'

Carl grinned, patted me on the back, pushed his jockey cap to the back of his curly ginger thatch and reeled off the latest news of our mutual acquaintances. Becky had gone home to Baltimore and would write soon. Karen seemed a little better and had been joined by her boyfriend from London, 'a real nice guy, although I don't understand half of what he says,' Carl admitted. Guy and Barbara were about to return to Florida, complete with juicer and good intentions. He himself was fine, just fine, tumour stationary, neither growing nor shrinking. 'What about you, Bee?' he asked. 'You look good, your colour has improved, but you don't look too happy. What's bothering you?'

'Just about everything . . . I think I'm going mad,' I said and went on to describe my weird rages and loss of control, half expecting Carl to make some bland, non-committal remark and then avoid me for ever after. 'It's not like me at all,' I said. 'I hate the way I've been carrying on, but there it is, I've hit an all-time low and I don't know how to get out of it.'

Carl shook his head and smiled. 'You needn't do anything. It'll go away, just like your diabetes did, remember? Please don't worry,' he said as calmly as if I had just been complaining about a gnat bite and not a total collapse of my normal value system and self-image. 'You're not going mad, you're just being detoxified. Have you forgotten? As the toxins leave the body, they affect the brain and the central nervous system and that's enough to drive you bananas. If you look it up in the book . . .'

'I've already done so,' I said. 'It's on page two hundred and two. Bad mood and depression is all it mentions, which is not the same as murderous rage and hatred. Besides, even the bad mood is supposed to be a by-product of a flare-up, and I haven't had one!'

'Never mind,' Carl said. 'Never mind. Keep your cool. We all get these dreadful moods and fits of rage sooner or later, with or without other symptoms. I've had them several times myself. They're all part of the process. Don't worry, they'll pass.'

'Well, if you say so.'

Maggie skipped out of her office across the courtyard.

She was smiling broadly and seemed to dance rather than walk as she came towards us. 'I'll take you to your quarters,' she said to Carl, 'but don't bother to unpack – tomorrow we're moving to the seaside, to the new clinic! I can hardly wait. We must be packed and ready to leave after lunch, so that there's no interruption in the juices. Two girls from the kitchen are going ahead to set up everything for the three o'clock liver juice. You'll see, we'll be much happier there.'

That afternoon I climbed up the steep hillside to my usual perch for the last time. Sitting quite still and letting my eyes drink in the wide view, I noted that my anger was settling down and beginning to ebb away. Toxins rushing through the brain and nervous system – yes, no doubt, but was that really all? I did not think so. Something else had also been at work: something old and powerful was bursting free with a vengeance. Could it be that the physical detoxification had a non-physical counterpart and that the cleansing of the body set off another, less obvious process of purification?

The invisible songbirds were calling to each other. I looked at my watch. It was time to trot back to La Mesa for another juice, another enema.

13

LIKE A BAND OF raggle-taggle gypsies, we moved from Clinic La Mesa to Clinic Del Sol in a small convoy of overloaded cars, trucks, campers and trailers, with patients, luggage, carrots and apples, equipment, files and everything else bundled together in organised disarray. Most of us were in high spirits. The total chaos of moving house made a stimulating break from our normal split-second, regulated routine. Tiny old Laetitia drove along in her own large car, which was just as well, because her enormous wardrobe would not have fitted into any of the communal vehicles; she had enough clothes to take her through the social seasons of several world capitals. Although she sometimes referred to herself as 'this child', she seemed complex and mysterious. The Christian fundamentalists recited their usual loud prayers before setting off and the woman missionary played a rousing tune on her accordion. It struck me that for a group of advanced cancer patients we were remarkably sturdy and mobile.

Clinic Del Sol turned out to be a converted motel, overlooking the Pacific but separated from it by a busy highway and an expanse of scrubby wasteland. The building was similar to La Mesa, with no garden, only a grassy back yard and some flowering trees outside the ground floor windows. It stood roughly in the middle of Playas de Tijuana, a long, narrow coastal resort or seaside suburb of no obvious charm or interest. 'I'm surprised we're allowed to stay so close to the ocean,' Carl said teasingly. 'After all, seawater is full of salt!'

'Ah yes,' Doris chimed in, 'that's why we mustn't swim in the sea or go to the beach – we might inhale too much salty air and suffer a setback.'

'Personally, I'll suffer a setback if I can't go down to the beach,' I said, too quietly to be heard. In the February sunshine the Pacific looked like the essence of blueness and radiance. I was perfectly happy to trade in that dusty hillside above La Mesa for the endless scintillating ocean view below Del Sol, and I could hardly wait to sneak down to the water's edge.

The clinic was ready for us, but the workmen had not yet removed the jazzy neon signs betraying its former existence as a motel, so that the front of this latest Gerson establishment still promised BAR PIZZAS COLOR TV and OPEN to all and sundry, although the first three items were no longer available and the fourth was no longer true. My room was smallish and dull, but at least it was all my own. I noted with relief that Maggie had put Tom and Lily into a double room at the opposite end of the building. I lay down on the bed with a sigh of contentment. I was feeling peaceful and in control, but after that shattering ten-day confrontation with my rage and darkness I now monitored my inner states gingerly, wondering whether there were any more ravening beasts hiding among the innocent foliage.

I tried to talk to Dr Arturo about the infantile, almost psychopathic violence of my anger but, like Carl, he regarded it as a detoxification symptom and attached no importance to it. He showed more interest when I told him that my old appendectomy scar had turned hot, red and painful. 'You see, that's another old injury being mended by the body,' he said. 'There's no need to do anything, just keep an eye on it; the scar will go back to normal once the repair is complete. I see you also have quite a few spots on your face. Excellent!'

'Is it? I find these spots appalling. They remind me of my adolescence which was one long skin eruption, the way I remember it. But then at least I had my whole

224

adult life to look forward to. Now I only get the spots without becoming young again. Tough, don't you think?'

But Dr Arturo was not to be drawn into frivolous exchanges. 'The appearance of the spots means,' he told me, 'that your organs of elimination are working flat out and even so they can't cope with all the toxins churned up in your body by the juices and the food; that's why some of it comes out through the skin. Be glad it's happening. It's a very good sign.'

'All right,' I said humbly. 'I'll try to be glad. But if I must have spots, I wish they'd appear elsewhere. On my bottom, for instance, where no one could see them.' (My wish was granted within forty-eight hours; unfortunately the spots on my face stayed put as well.) 'I also wish my tumour didn't bulge so much. I can't help feeling that it's still growing.'

'No, it isn't. Please believe me, it isn't. But there's some swelling around it and that makes it look bigger. Also, the lump has become more movable, which is good.' He gave me a patient, resigned look. 'You've been here for just over five weeks now and you've produced no further tumours beyond the one you arrived with. Yet with metastasized melanoma you would have grown quite a few if the therapy hadn't gained some measure of control over the malignant process. We have a melanoma patient at La Gloria,' he went on, 'who's had two secondary tumours removed from her neck before coming to us . . . and another two popped up even before the surgical incision had healed. I know of another one who produced a total of fifty tumours in five months. That's the speed of your type of cancer. But you have only one tumour. I can only repeat, you're doing well and you'd do even better if you stopped worrying.'

I nodded. He was right. I simply had to find more trust and steadfastness in myself. In the light of what was at stake, my current symptoms – a dry mouth, grogginess, fits of palpitation – were almost too trivial to mention. I did ask though how long I would have to go on taking castor oil every other day, and was told that the minimum period was three months; after that I would have to take it twice a week for eight months, and then once a week until further notice. Ugh, ugh. I had a brief vision of a set of clean, clear, pure guts, as bright as stainless steel; then I remembered the dull, heavy, viscous castor oil and its dreadful aftertaste on the tongue. Ugh, ugh. But I knew better than to argue. Besides, it was not a matter of arguing with some outside authority. Dr Arturo gave instructions, but it was up to me whether I followed them. Oddly enough, this very freedom acted on me like a strong discipline. I knew that I would have to go on taking the wretched castor oil, even at home where there would be no muscular Mexican maids handing it to me and watching, with unmalicious glee, while I swallowed it.

'Let me see your skin graft, please,' Dr Arturo said. It was a routine inspection, but this time, as he ran his fingertips over the ugly, pared-to-the-bone area, I uttered a yelp of surprise. 'No, no, it doesn't hurt,' I cried, 'it's only that I could feel your touch. For the first time since the operation the skin graft has . . . responded!' We looked at each other, I in a state of great excitement, he with a slow smile spreading over his face. 'Until now,' I explained, 'whenever you touched the graft, I felt absolutely nothing, it was completely numb, like a piece of marble. But now – '

He ran his fingertips across and beyond the graft two or three times. 'Does the graft feel the same as the rest of your leg?'

'Oh no, it doesn't,' I said, 'the sensation is much weaker in the graft, but at least some response has returned. I suppose the nerves are beginning to grow back.' There were tears in my eyes. I felt as if my martyred and alienated limb had been partly restored to me.

'You see?' Dr Arturo said, with only the gentlest hint of reproach. I nodded tearfully. 'I shouldn't be surprised,' he added, 'if some of the flesh and fat regrew on that leg. It would be highly unusual and it may never happen, but it's not impossible.' He smiled and departed, leaving me in a state of joyful amazement. And even though two days later Charlotte regretfully but firmly discounted Dr Arturo's forecast, saying that my leg was far too damaged to be able to rebuild itself, I did not feel unhappy. The fact that some nerve contact had been re-established between Mr Lennox's senseless handiwork and the rest of me seemed almost miraculous, somewhat like a dry, dead branch bursting into leaf. Welcome back, I said to the formerly dead part of my right leg; you were away a long time.

To celebrate I crept out of the clinic, crossed the roaring highway and walked down an unpaved road towards the sea. What attracted me was a brilliant green grove of luxuriant trees and shrubs by the water's edge, an emerald oasis rising from a desert of dry earth and pale weeds. But as I hurried towards it, I was abruptly stopped by a terrible stench that rose in front of me like a wall. That gorgeous vegetation, I now saw, was growing in and around a sewage works built on the shore, and built so inefficiently that foul-smelling waste water was oozing from it in all directions. Paradise found and instantly lost, I thought regretfully. How ironical to find such an installation on my very first outing, as if the enema bucket were not enough to focus my mind on matters of sewage.

Well, that green grove had to be avoided. I continued along the coastal path, looking for a suitable perch from which to contemplate the sea. Playas de Tijuana seemed to be on the crest of a building boom. Countless small square houses, half built or newly completed, stood between the coast and the hills, forming random patterns as if they had been scattered by a careless giant or a mad architect. Tan, orange, pink, green, ox-blood red

227

and white houses rose everywhere from the compacted grey soil which did not look as if it could sustain even the few spindly plants struggling for life in minute front gardens. The unpaved roads were of the kind that blow away in dry weather and drown you in mud when the rains come. Torn posters on walls and lamp-posts advertised dance bands and politicians. A handful of graffiti celebrated PUNKS DE LA COSTA, proving that at least one British export had reached this alien shore. The scene was flat and dismal yet overlaid with glitter, for there was broken glass everywhere, both large, jagged pieces and finely ground fragments of green, brown and white, sparkling and winking in the dirt. The place was an environmentalist's nightmare; plundered, exploited, disfigured; a piece of earth that seemed to have no friends. For a brief angry moment I suspected that half the population spent part of its time breaking glass and scattering it, while the other half filled up the empty spaces with flattened beer cans.

Eventually I found a deserted spot behind a large building, a gentle slope with the remains of concrete steps leading down to the stony beach. I sat down on a crumbling step halfway down the slope, screened from the road by a patch of fuzzy weeds, and surrendered to the view. *Thalassa*, the sea, there it was again, blue and endless, swaying, dancing, rocking, pounding forth its rhythm. Above all, reminding.

If my experience of cancer has any meaning, I thought, if there is more to it than what I can see here and now, let me get it right. The long waves advanced and retreated. Far out, two or three misty humps rose from the horizon, islands I would never visit. To the right, towards the US border, a helicopter patrolled the skies, looking for would-be illegal immigrants. The concrete step made an uncomfortable perch, but I decided to visit it every afternoon in order to stretch my soul and exercise my legs, strictly in that order. For a few moments I had a strange sensation of the inner and

228

the outer, the experience and the meaning, the detail and the outline meeting and merging within me, creating a sense of wholeness that made my heart sing. Then the sensation faded and I walked back to the clinic.

'Just read this,' Carl said later that afternoon, handing me an article clipped from an American medical journal.

'Malignant melanoma is one of the most unpredictable cancers,' the piece began and went on to say that if the disease remained limited to the original site, the chances of surviving five years after aggressive surgery were about seventy per cent. 'On the other hand,' I read, 'if the cancer has spread beyond the original site to the regional lymph glands, such as under the arm or in the groin, the five-year survival rate drops to about twenty per cent.' We exchanged a glance. Neither of us seemed perturbed.

'Depressing,' I said, 'except that these figures refer to conventionally treated sufferers and so they aren't relevant to Gerson patients. Do you know,' I added with a sudden burst of gaiety, 'we are a most conscious group of patients. We not only know what we've got and take responsibility for our treatment, we even consult the medical literature to keep up to date with the gloom and doom discoveries. Whether we'll recover or not, at least we face reality.'

'What do you mean, whether we'll recover or not? How often do I have to tell you that we'll be okay, especially because we're not frightened? Get that into your head, Bee, otherwise I won't lend you any more depressing literature,' Carl said and sauntered back to his room. He kept a large seed tray outside his door, full of luxuriant wheatgrass, a highly valued item in the alternative diet field, since fresh wheatgrass juice has been found to be the nearest thing in composition to healthy human blood. Visitors to Carl's room were encouraged to pick and chew a few blades. The grass yielded a sweet, powerful juice and then had to be discarded, for the fibrous part did not break down,

229

however long we chewed it. While Carl grew wheat-grass, other patients used large jars to sprout lentils, mung beans and alfalfa seeds which they added to their salads and soups. Sprouted seeds were good sources of vegetable protein, enzymes and other live substances. We already consumed them in our green juices, but all that supplementary indoor farming was part of the patients' preparations for surviving at home where they would have to grow their own supplies, with help from the clinic staff. Ah yes, going home. I decided to do that exactly two months after my arrival, on the 20th March which happened to coincide with the spring equinox and the full moon; an auspicious day, I thought, for starting a new chapter. That left me another twenty-two days at the clinic, which in gut-clock terms equalled one hundred and ten enemas and eleven doses of castor oil; or, at a slightly higher level, two hundred and eighty-six juices.

At least these were quantities I could imagine and handle. My sense of time, however, behaved erratically. On the one hand I was sharply aware of how every day took me closer to home; on the other, time had lost all shape and meaning, so that every now and then it felt as if my stay at Del Sol might go on for ever. Fortunately, Hudie's letters reminded me of the wider world outside the therapy, and this provided some structure to existence. He wrote almost every day, which for a confirmed non-correspondent of his kind was a supreme feat. I gathered from his letters that he was gradually assembling a Gerson mini-clinic in my house, installing the juicing equipment, setting up the organic vegetable and liver supplies, negotiating with a pro-spective daily help and keeping my friends supplied with news. Hudie, I thought, with enormous gratitude, was life's consolation for everything that had gone wrong in the past few decades. Without his help I would not have even considered attempting the therapy at home. And I was not sure whether even with his help I would be able to cope.

I had barely got over the way in which my skin graft was now responding to touch when my body produced another sign of regeneration. It started modestly enough. One morning, when the regular maid brought along my breakfast, I detected a faint whiff of violet-scented toilet water around her. Two or three days later I was surprised to notice that she had switched to a stronger version of the same scent. After another two days her aura of violets became almost overpowering, as if she had deliberately progressed from a feeble *eau de toilette* to a concentrated scent. Somehow that did not seem likely, nor did the girl's choice of scent concern me, except that something at the back of my mind kept returning to this puzzling escalation of violets. At last I found the likely answer. The girl had been wearing the same scent all along; it was my sense of smell that had been growing stronger and clearer every day, until the previously faint aura began to register as a powerful odour.

To test my hypothesis, I went round the clinic sniffing and picking up scents like a truffle hound getting into practice after a long rest, and I found that my nose was unmistakably sharper than before, possibly as sharp as it had been in childhood. This was exciting. I went to the kitchen, ostensibly to watch the juice-making, but in fact testing my nose in the many-flavoured atmosphere. Two girls were scrubbing mountains of carrots and apples, one was stirring a cauldronful of the pungent Hippocrates soup, another one was chopping onions and peeling garlic, and as I stood watching them, I was astounded by the sharpness and purity of all those smells as they hit my nose separately and in chorus. The experience was extraordinary. It was the olfactory version of seeing no longer through a glass darkly but face to face. I recalled Charlotte's stories about patients regaining their hearing or recovering much of their eyesight as a by-product of the therapy; obviously detoxification also helped to improve the sense of smell. I was delighted with this latest spin-off of the therapy, even though I realised that it would also intensify the impact of bad smells.

I soon noticed that my other senses were also functioning better, but I had no obvious yardstick, comparable to the maid's violet scent, with which to measure the gradual change. But at least now I understood that it was my improved hearing that made the kitchen staff sound noisier every day, and enabled me to listen to the radio with the volume control at its lowest setting. I also realised why my left eye, always the weaker of the two, had no more focussing problems. It was terrific, this gradual repair and restoration of my senses, and also its promise of wider implications. Surely, if ridding the body of accumulated toxins could achieve the apparently impossible task of restoring middle-aged sense organs to an almost youthful degree of functioning, then perhaps other ravages of the ageing process could also be made good. Perhaps the reason why so many recovered Gerson patients remained hale and active well into their eighties was because their altered lifestyle stopped their bodies from getting silted up with waste matter. Was ageing basically a slow poisoning of the system, in which the clogged and overloaded organs eventually broke down in a variety of ways? I remembered the case of Dr Albert Schweitzer who at the age of seventy-five consulted Dr Gerson about his advanced diabetes and depression, was cured by him within a short time and went on working in Africa until he was over ninety.

I was pondering the matter under a sunshade on the terrace – we had strict instructions to keep out of the strong sunshine – when I realised that at least one answer was there, under my very nose. An old couple, whom I had often observed, were emerging from their room into the bright courtyard. Flora, the wife, was suffering from Alzheimer's disease, a distressing form of senility accompanied by double incontinence, loss of speech, memory and movement, and deep lethargy. Flora was seventy-seven, white-haired, with large, unhappy dark eyes. Her husband Mario was six years older; he was sturdy and vigorous and totally devoted to his wife. He always held her hand, never let her out of his sight and made sure that she got enough exercise by walking her up and down, around and around, slowly, patiently; and Flora shuffled along on her thin legs and uncertain feet, like a miserable ancient child with nothing to say for herself.

Except that she was beginning to talk a little. She had visibly improved even since I had been watching her. Her movements were more co-ordinated, her posture less droopy. Yes, she was progressing well, said her daughter Joy when I asked her about her mother's condition. Flora had been brought to the clinic on a stretcher in a catatonic state, unable to stand, let alone walk. In one month she had regained a good deal of mobility, bowel control, some speech, and even the first twinklings of memory. 'She's getting quite lively for short spells,' Joy added. 'Yesterday she ticked off my father and got angry with me – we were so glad to see her snap out of her lethargy. But what a hard business this treatment is!'

Joy and her man, Roger, lived in a motor camper which they parked in the clinic's backyard. They had given up their usual nomadic existence for a while in order to help look after Flora. 'It's too much for my father,' Joy explained. 'He's eighty-three and set in his ways, but he wants my mother to get well. The drug treatment she was given before we came here made her worse, and there's no other alternative.' She saw that the therapy brought results but did not agree with it entirely. As a strict vegetarian she disliked the idea of liver juices and injections. As a confirmed raw food eater she thought patients were given too much cooked food to eat. Above all, like myself, she worried about the total absence of psychological back-up at the clinic – no counselling, no one to teach relaxation, yoga, meditation or visualisation. How were patients to rebalance their lives towards health if all the care and effort were concentrated on their bodies? I sighed and told her about my old dream of finding the modern equivalent of a holistic Greek healing sanctuary, and how the dream had receded under the pressure of physical chores and inner upheavals. 'If you can't find your sanctuary, you'll have to found one yourself,' she said. It was a nice thought, but I could not and did not take it seriously.

Joy was gentle, intuitive and unconventional, a late-flowering rebel who had dropped out of middle-class affluence in early middle-age and was now seeking her salvation in various alternative and esoteric fields. During my last two weeks at the clinic I spent much time with her and Roger, a tall, blond Viking who made some of the short, dark Mexican maids giggle and sigh behind his back. Sometimes Carl joined us; sometimes we sat with Flora and Mario, pumping conversation, interest and energy into the old lady, responding to her incomplete questions as well as we could. As I watched Flora gradually moving away from the edge of hopeless senility, I could not help seeing her as a guinea-pig for other stricken old people, just as I saw myself in the same role in the cancer field. Exactly how our experiences were to be utilised and made available to others was not at all clear.

The image I still carry of Joy and Roger from our brief period of concentrated friendship is the one I used to see every morning from my window. There was Joy sitting on a patch of grass in the backyard, meditating in the lotus position, her straw hat tilted forward to shut out the world, her cloud of dark hair covering her shoulders like a fur collar. Roger sat a few feet away. Sometimes he played his small, lute-shaped African instrument that had metal strips for strings and issued a soft, monotonous, infinitely gentle tune that was itself a kind of meditation. Between the two of them they produced a quality of stillness and peace that was almost tangible. I knew its flavour, even though for the time being it remained inaccessible.

Even so, I was comforted by a dream, a single solitary dream that had somehow managed to break through into waking consciousness. In it an unknown woman showed me a vast spiral of brilliant stars, rising in ever-wider circles into infinity; some people, she said, mistook it for the Milky Way. No more was said, but I was transfixed by the power of the image.

Around this time Mike, the gloomy Dane, began to spend more time lying fully dressed on his bed, watching his portable TV set and taking his meals in his room. Laetitia tried to reactivate him and gave him a good talking-to on the need for effort and commitment to the therapy, but told us afterwards that Mike seemed apathetic and unwilling to stir. 'Why, he's even cut down on the castor oil,' she said indignantly. 'He says he doesn't like it – God Almighty, does anyone *like* it? I don't think he understands what he's supposed to be doing. Little wonder he's getting worse.' We hummed and hawed anxiously. Phyllis, our chief source of rumours and gossip, dropped her voice to intimate that Mike had been breaking the rules all along, but however hard we grilled her, she refused to go into details. Eventually, Mike's younger brother arrived for a visit. He was large and taciturn, and although he ate with us in the dining-room, he did not indicate what he thought about the clinic or the treatment; and after two days of non-communication he simply disappeared, taking Mike with him. They departed swiftly and quietly, without a word to anyone, without leaving a message or an address, and although none of us had had any real contact with Mike, we all felt sad and disturbed, as if a death had occurred among us.

On the same day, after dinner, the kitchen staff invited us all to a baby shower, held for a very pregnant maid who was about to stop work. The mother-to-be sat heavily but happily in the middle, receiving useful gifts from her workmates, while Luis the cook danced around with his flashlight camera, taking pictures from every angle. The radio played smouldering jazz. The staff shared a bright blue cake decorated with baby dolls; we were offered huge helpings of fresh fruit salad. It was a noisy, happy occasion, a kind of fertility celebration, and we patients, pregnant with our cancers, sat around benevolently, grateful to be there. In some irrational way the baby shower softened the shock of Mike's disappearance.

Now that my time at Del Sol was running out, I launched myself into a final bout of reading, borrowing every available book on alternative medicine and allied subjects. I started with Book One of the Essene Gospel of Peace, recommended by Charlotte. To my amazement it turned out to be a Biblical guide to an early version of the Gerson therapy. It is the story of how Jesus teaches a crowd of sick and maimed people to make themselves whole again by eating vegetarian food, avoiding toxins (known as 'abominations'), cleansing their bodies and even giving themselves enemas, with the aid of 'a large trailing gourd, having a stalk the length of a man,' suitably hollowed out. The teaching also contains a recipe for making bread from sprouted grain and baking it in the heat of the sun. Oddly enough the only bread served at the clinic was Essene bread, made in California according to that same recipe (although we suspected that it had been baked in an oven).

The Essene Gospel was more radical than the Gerson therapy in its opposition to cooked food: 'Eat not anything which fire, or frost, or water has destroyed,' says Jesus, praising the virtues of a raw diet. That one difference apart, the similarity between the Essene therapy and ours was startlingly close. But when I expressed my delight over this, I was slapped down by one of the Christian fundamentalists. 'That book is a fake and a forgery,' he declared in the tones of an angry prophet. 'If I were you, I'd have nothing to do with it.' And when I asked him why he disliked it so much, he became even angrier. 'Can you imagine,' he asked me, 'Our Lord discussing *enemas* with the multitudes?' Why yes, I could, and in fact I preferred the idea of a practical, holistic, healing Jesus to that of an ethereal, incompletely embodied theoretician; to my mind, official Christianity's uneasy, rejecting attitude to the body was almost blasphemous and a major source of pain and failure among the faithful; but I chose to keep quiet. Across the border in California the Evolutionists and Creationists were already fighting yet another battle; I had no wish to introduce a theological argument into the dining-room of Del Sol.

Still I went on reading: books, brochures and articles on the healing power of clay, on all-fruit diets, on indoor farming and, above all, on the importance of a healthy colon, a subject on which most schools of thought seemed to agree. 'There is no disease, only a polluted body,' I read in a far-out book on nature cure. 'Death is the unknown in which all of us lived before birth,' I read in a Zen-flavoured book by Alan Watts. 'It should be forbidden and severely punished to remove cancer by cutting, burning, cautery and other fiendish torture,' I read the words of Paracelsus, the sixteenth century physician – 'it is from nature that the disease arises and from nature comes the cure, not from the physician.' I read avidly, as if trying to lay in stocks of information for the lean times to come. Back home, I thought, I might have very little leisure for reading.

Carl brought over his car from San Diego and organised an expedition to the Tijuana craft market, where a vast medley of largely ghastly souvenirs included portraits of Elvis Presley machine-embroidered in silver on black, hand-painted plaster figures of Botticelli's Venus, and small versions of Rodin's Lovers in a pose that went well beyond the limits intended by the sculptor. But I searched on, determined to take back some keepsake, and eventually bought a pottery cat and an owl made of jute, which I recognised only much later as those eternal lovers, the Owl and the Pussy-Cat. I also had a haircut in a cavernous salon in Tijuana, where holy pictures of the Madonna, her heart pierced by seven knives, alternated with large photographs of bare breasts and thighs, advertising a French body lotion; an original way, I thought, of reconciling two aspects of womanhood. My hair was now a mixture of brown, beige, grey and white, like the fleece of some hopelessly confused sheep. Poor Hudie, I thought, getting me back with the spotty, blotchy face of an aged adolescent underneath a variegated thatch of badly cut hair – he deserves something better than that. But then, I thought, at least he is getting me back alive.

On my last Saturday at the clinic I listened to Charlotte's weekly talk in a mood of leave-taking. She sounded sombre as she described the worsening health picture in the industrialised West, with degenerative diseases striking at an earlier age in each succeeding generation. The link between cause and effect was clear, but no one in a position of power chose to act on it, so that the built-in faults of the Western lifestyle remained uncorrected. Child diabetes in the US was rising by six per cent a year, but the average canned baby food still contained up to twenty per cent of sugar. Cancer was the second biggest killer among the under-eighteens, straight after accidents, but the medical profession went on tinkering with its high technology gadgets instead of denouncing the lifestyle that produced cancer. 'This year,' she said, 'seven hundred and eighty-five thousand Americans are expected to get cancer. We're reaching the stage when one in four people will get the disease. In 1936 the ratio was one in fourteen. Yet five

238

years ago, in 1976, when the US Senate Committee on nutritional needs and health suggested a reduced intake of salt, sugar, meat and processed foods,' she went on, her voice taking on a bitter edge, 'the American Medical Association rejected those recommendations, claiming that there was no evidence to link diet and disease. You won't be surprised to hear that the booklet containing the Senate Committee's findings is no longer available.'

I watched her with affection and sadness. She was so brave and seemed so alone, fighting every inch of the way, with no hope of winning against the mammoths of orthodoxy, vested interests and entrenched power structures. But then it occurred to me that perhaps the real changes would erupt at grassroots level, on a self-help basis; and if they did, I wanted to be there to help them along.

'I'm afraid this is goodbye,' I said to Charlotte after her lecture. 'I'll be flying home in five days and shan't see you again before then. Thanks for everything. I'll miss you – things will be tough in London.'

'Well, my daughter Margaret is there, she'll help you when you get stuck.'

'Oh, I know that. But there'll be no clinic to flee to if things get awkward. Quite frankly, I'm scared.'

'That's quite normal. Most patients are scared when they go home from here. It's like cutting the umbilicus all over again. The first few weeks will be tough, but then you should find your feet. Anyway, do you realise how much better you look now than when you arrived? There's no comparison. I know that your tumour hasn't shrunk, but that doesn't matter; it may turn into a harmless dead mass without ever shrinking in size. No need to worry as long as it doesn't grow bigger or sprout further lumps.'

I nodded. 'Agreed. What worries me though is that I didn't have a single flare-up in two months, although I've had just about everything else.'

'I'm sorry about that,' Charlotte said. 'Some patients

239

start late, a tiny minority even get well without flare-ups, but I do think you'll have yours in due course. Besides, by now you know what to do when you get a reaction, don't you? Of course you do. You'll be all right.'

She warned me about the inconvenience of the long flight home, with no chance of an enema for fifteen or sixteen hours, which could be quite a shock to the rapidly detoxifying system, used to regular cleansing five times a day; not long enough to cause liver coma, but potentially a major nuisance. She also urged me not to accept any airline refreshments. 'You're at a stage when convenience foods full of salt and chemicals would upset your system badly,' she explained. 'Maggie will give you some food for your flight. If you run out, fast rather than eat junk.'

We shook hands. I saw her to her car and waved as she drove off towards La Gloria. From the sharp sense of loss I experienced at that moment I realised how much I had come to rely on Charlotte for support and reassurance, almost expecting her to win my battles for me. This was the diffident, dependent, orphaned inner child coming to the surface again, looking for a magical adult to take things over, produce a cure, kill the dragon or, rather, the monster crab, cause the sun to shine. Poor Charlotte, I thought, what a load of projections patients must be putting on her, as if she did not have enough burdens to bear. But then perhaps she was too busy battling with her work to notice how some of us were turning her into a universal Great Mother, possessor of all the answers. The kindest thing I could do for her was to withdraw my projections and learn to stand on my own two feet once more.

On my last evening at Del Sol I sat down on my bed to examine my right leg which had been feeling alarmingly tight for several days, tight to the point of pain. As I looked at it, I noticed to my amazement that a small piece of new flesh had grown underneath the upper right side of the skin graft, nestling like a soft, live cushion at the edge of that pared-to-the-bone disaster area. Not quite believing my eyes, I touched it again and again until there could be no doubt that by the eighth week of the therapy my slaughtered leg had begun to rebuild itself. You are clever, I said inwardly to my body; even Charlotte did not think you could do it. Personally I would be happier if you started getting rid of the tumour instead of mending the leg, but of course you must follow your own priorities.

I was overjoyed and awed by this strange development. Clearly my body had unsuspected self-healing powers and a kind of independent wisdom that moved into action as soon as conditions were right. This was a physical vindication of the old Raja yoga aphorism, 'Remove the obstacle and the result will appear.' Who could tell what other tricks and small miracles this far from dumb body was capable of?

It was getting late. My bags were packed. Joy dropped in for a final talk. We walked down to the nearest headland and listened to the sea. It sounded deep and rich and for a moment reminded me of the voice of the night sea just off Ithaka, as heard from a becalmed boat. Wily Odysseus, I thought, here we go again, off on another voyage; keep an eye on me.

14

ON MY LAST morning at Del Sol my thermometer rolled off the table for no obvious reason and broke into smithereens on the floor. That small event left me as startled as the spontaneous disintegration of my BBC identity disc had done three months earlier. I seemed to be unable to end a phase without some symbolic object committing ritual suicide to mark the occasion. Luckily, I had plenty of new, non-symbolic objects to launch me into the next phase. A large crate in the corner contained enough medication for six months, including syringes and needles for the liver injections (which Maggie had taught me to self-administer), sets of closely woven juice cloths, a box of herb tea with a strong anti-cancer reputation, and a packet of therapeutic clay for poultices. Heaven alone knew what HM Customs Officer at Gatwick airport was going to make of that lot.

Before vacating my room I sat down for a moment to assess my situation. It was now almost three months since I had broken away from Lennox and the orthodoxy he stood for. That meant that I had used up three out of the six months he had given me as my maximum life expectancy if I refused surgery. (The minimum, that of six weeks, had passed long ago.) I was not only alive but also much better in every way, free of diabetes and arthritis and apparently able to grow back at least part of my mutilated right leg. Above all, I still had no more than the one solitary tumour I had arrived with, instead of the dreaded proliferation of lumps that was usual with melanoma. All that meant that so far the therapy had been working well in its quiet, unsensational way. So far, so good, touch wood. But I told myself that I must not get over-confident and commit the fatal mistake of some Gerson patients who, emboldened by their rapid improvement, loosened up their daily routine and paid dearly for it. No, over-confidence was out. True, my life felt cramped in the straitjacket of the regime, densely body-centred and fragmented, but that was a reasonable price to pay for being alive. I had developed a certain toughness and single-mindedness in confronting the task in hand. At least for the time being the balance sheet was in my favour.

My final round of farewells proved to be oddly poignant, even in the case of patients whom I did not like. Since our collective prospects were uncertain, I felt uneasy about breaking up our shared pattern by removing myself from it, and of course my separation anxiety added to the apprehension I felt. Suddenly the clinic seemed to be the only safe spot in the world where survival was possible, though not guaranteed; was I making a dreadful mistake in leaving it?

Seen for the last time through those jumbled feelings, even the least attractive patients seemed acceptable. And when I got round to the ones I liked, I found I did not want to leave them at all. I sat for a while in a half-darkened room with Doris, the black ex-nurse who had been in bed for several days, feeling unwell. 'Thank you for setting me such high standards,' I said to her. 'You're always beautifully turned out, with your hair perfectly done, so that every time I felt like letting myself go, you made me pull myself together simply by being around. That's been a great help.'

Doris opened her eyes wide. 'Okay, I like nice clothes,' she said with a chuckle, 'but what do you mean about my hair? I thought everybody knew that I wore a wig; how else would I have such straight, smooth hair? Still, I'm pleased if I helped to keep up your morale. The problem is to keep up my own.' Even in the half-light I could see a thin white hairline beneath her black one, where the pillow had slightly dislocated her wig. This made me sad, as if a chink had been opened in her defences. We shook hands. Her skin felt cold and clammy. Before leaving I offered to raise her blind to let in the gentle spring sunlight, but she declined. Her eyes, she said, were tired, just like the rest of her.

Laetitia received me in a state of regal ill temper, certainly not in the mood for anything as downbeat as saying goodbye. She treated me to a blistering attack on orthodox doctors in general and cancer specialists in particular; she declared that our diet was too alkaline and very bad for her fingernails; she showed me an exquisite miniature still life she had created out of leaves, pebbles and strategically placed drops of water; and, as an afterthought, she commanded me to convey her greetings to Europe. I watched her with awe and love. There was real fire in her tiny old body, together with the kind of ultimate courage that knows how to ignore tiresome things like frailty, loneliness and an increasingly alien world. 'I should be painting in Greece right now,' she said crossly, 'instead of sitting here and going crazy with boredom.' With a bit of luck, I suggested, she would soon be well enough to leave for home and get out her palette for a practice run. Oh yes, of course, she agreed with queenly nonchalance, plenty of time to go to Greece; and then she bade me to take good care of my colon. Under the circumstances that was as good a valediction as any.

With Carl the farewell was brief – he was just about to drive to La Gloria on some private business. We stood in the courtyard near one of the flowering trees which were regularly visited by humming-birds. I took a last look at his thin frame and shrewd, sardonic face framed in curly ginger hair and realised that although we had spent many hours discussing a great variety of subjects, ranging from Christ's divinity to the best way of making fatless yogurt, we did not know each other at all. I did not even know his age – late thirties? – or what he did for a living, and could no more imagine his existence outside the clinic than he could imagine mine. Yet we had had a good, close comradeship, bonded by our shared disease, and that had been a great gift to me. 'I know what you're going to tell me,' I now said, 'but this time let me say it to you. We're going to make it, you and I, we're going to get well, there's simply no doubt about it.'

He grinned and shook my hand. 'Absolutely correct, Bee,' he said. 'I'm glad you've learned it at last – at one stage I didn't think you would, with all those doubts of yours. Just work hard at it when you're at home. It's not easy, I can tell you that. Well, if you'll pardon me, I'll be off now – I don't like goodbyes.' He got into his car and drove off, stirring up a cloud of dust outside the clinic's back gate.

Maggie handed me my provisions: two thermos flasks filled with apple and carrot juice, fresh fruit, a chunk of Essene bread and a couple of cold jacket potatoes. It seemed very little for such a long flight, but the clinic's driver was anxious for us to leave and I did not want to cause a delay. 'Please remember to hold the needle straight when you give yourself the liver jab,' Maggie said by way of farewell; she had trained me thoroughly in the art of self-injecting but obviously was not sure that I had got it right. Other familiar faces swam in and out of view, calling out greetings and good wishes.

'Let's go,' I said to the driver, 'before it gets too emotional for me.'

Adios, keep well, see ya, Godspeed. We were off, heading for the US border. The Pacific shone like a silver mirror.

The American frontier guard was not interested in my visa and did not stamp my passport. He did, however, search my luggage for Laetrile, the controversial anti-cancer substance which I did not possess. I said so repeatedly, but I might not have spoken. After the laissez-faire atmosphere of Mexico his square-jawed officiousness seemed particularly silly. 'Take no notice of him,' the driver said after we had entered the US. 'These guys know me by sight, they know that I ferry patients to and from San Diego. What they don't know is that our patients hardly ever take Laetrile. But then they don't know the difference between our clinic and the others, those of Kelley, Hoxsey, Contreras and so on; to them it's all part of the Tijuana cancer belt and all they want to find is Laetrile.' I nodded. It did not really matter. After the dust and aridity of Mexico, California was a lush Garden of Eden. One day, I thought, I would like to come back and plant a tree belt around Tijuana.

The full weight of my loneliness hit me only after the driver had left me at San Diego airport. All right, I thought with a sinking heart, there is no more umbilicus to hang on to, I am on my own, better start functioning like an adult once more. After all, I had been an experienced practising adult before the therapy presented me with certain things that took me straight back to childhood – thin gruel, stewed fruit, camomile tea, castor oil, enemas, early bedtime, strict rules, obedience to the great absent father-figure of Dr Gerson, and, as the final criterion of childhood, total dependence on a system that had been there long before I arrived on the scene. Yet despite all that I was still able to masquerade as a grown-up.

I sat down in the departure lounge and watched the people milling around the place. At first it was great fun to see so many strangers after the limited number of familiar faces at the clinic, but when the novelty wore off, I was astonished to notice how unhealthy most of these strangers looked. With a few exceptions they were all overweight and also bent or lopsided, round-shouldered or plain shapeless, with pasty faces and dull eyes. The heavy make-up of the women startled me. So did the tension in so many faces. But the oddest thing was that most of these people were busy consuming something much of the time – peanuts, sweets or chewing gum, as if keeping their jaws still had been wrong or dangerous. They are all mad, I thought; somebody ought to tell them not to poison themselves with all that junk, you only have to look at them to see how unhealthy they are. And then I was overcome by the weird humour of the moment, for there I was, fresh from a cancer clinic, finding that the officially healthy, normal people inhabiting the outside world looked distinctly unwell compared to the seriously ill patients I had just left behind. We may be very ill but at least we look reasonably fit, I thought, savouring the absurdity of my observation, and our lifestyle is a hundred times healthier than the average person's. I must tell Hudie about this, I thought, it will make him laugh.

Hudie was now only some twelve hours away, counting from take-off at Los Angeles. He would be waiting for me at Gatwick, looking as solid and reassuring as ever, a man who knew how to deal with things. Above all, he would put an end to the loneliness of the past two months which I had not fully acknowledged until that moment, just as I had not allowed myself to think too much of my closest friends, for fear of getting too miserable. But all that was nearly over, I could drop my defences and relax into anticipation. I sighed with relief and drank some carrot juice.

My joy began to fade at Los Angeles airport where, for technical reasons, we were unable to take off at the scheduled time. The delay grew longer and longer, until at last we were carted off to a hotel for a meal. By now it was evening. I had used up my rations, my stomach was roaring for food, and so, disobeying Charlotte's instructions, I ate a mixed salad and some boiled potatoes. The food tasted awful and made me feel guilty.

Back at the airport, waiting in great discomfort, I experienced the anxiety of any patient whose vital therapeutic routine is broken. I suddenly knew what it must feel like to be a diabetic running out of insulin or a cardiac patient vainly looking for some life-saving tablets. I had no idea how long I would manage without juices, enemas and medication without my body going haywire. Charlotte had said that the long flight might cause problems; what extra complications was the delay adding to them? My excitement about going home had vanished. What I really wanted was to be back at the clinic.

At last, after several misleading announcements, we took off six hours late. Feeling weary, I told a hostess that I was ill and needed rest. She bedded me down across three empty seats and I dozed off at once. I woke up two hours later, feeling mortally ill. There seemed to be a hatchet embedded in the back of my skull. Every now and then the jagged blade shuddered and twisted, sending shafts of pain through my head. My stomach felt as if someone had turned it inside out and then filled it with toxic slush. The nausea was worse than anything I had experienced before – worse than my vilest seasickness on a long-ago voyage to Canada, worse even than the nearly fatal shellfish poisoning I had suffered in Marseilles. Waves of shivering alternated with heat, until the shivers stopped and I knew that I was running a very high temperature.

I lay there very still, very frightened, drained of strength, trying to make sense of my internal storm. What was going on? Was I by any chance dying? Had my cancer started an offensive on all fronts to make up for lost time? Was I sailing into a stroke – surely not with my low blood pressure – or into a heart attack? Had the hotel meal poisoned me?

One by one I considered every fatal condition I could think of, until I was struck by a wildly funny insight.

The only thing that was wrong with me was that I

had started my first flare-up, the one that was often the worst. Not having produced one in two months while being surrounded by the clinic's facilities and expert care, I was having it now, thousands of feet above the frozen wastes of Canada, stuck in a jumbo jet, with no hope of help, relief or escape. Honestly, I thought, of all the stupid and unsuitable places in the civilised world my body has chosen just about the worst for this exercise: I cannot get off the plane for a quick enema in Alaska or Labrador, yet that would be the only effective remedy; there is no gruel or peppermint tea within reach and I am stuck for at least another nine hours when I do not even know how to survive the next five minutes. I was familiar with life's little ironies, but this was going beyond a joke. Yet I could see the joke, too.

Virtue, as I had long suspected, was its own punishment. As long as I had rigorously followed the therapy, sticking to it both in letter and in spirit, the longed-for reward, namely a flare-up, had not materialised. But now that circumstances had forced me to break the rules, my body had promptly flung itself into a vigorous reaction, fulfilling my greatest wish – except that I was in no position to feel pleased about it.

As my sickness worsened, I lost the joke altogether. In the washroom mirror my face looked horribly yellow. Bile rampant, I thought. Instant jaundice. My liver is in trouble. The worst thing we had been warned about was happening. I staggered back to my improvised sofa. A hostess hurried across to ask if I wanted anything. I felt parched but did not dare to drink tea or coffee. She offered me fresh orange juice. I accepted. It was fresh out of a tin and my stomach promptly rejected it. Plain water went the same way. All right, no drink. A slow, low-key dimness was spreading through my brain. Was this the dreaded hepatic coma that had killed some of Dr Gerson's early patients for want of detoxification? No, probably just ordinary toxins streaming through the brain. Please God do not let me pass out. Why ever not? I wondered a moment later: if I passed out, I would not feel a thing.

If only I could get out of my skin, the next leaden thought rolled up. Or out of the aircraft. I squinted at the window above my head, willing it to open briefly so that I might be syphoned out, in the style of an old James Bond film, without affecting the other passengers. Nothing happened. Then a kindly mist spread inside my eyelids and I went to sleep.

At Gatwick I was dimly conscious of being helped up, straightened, put together and escorted down the gangway. No doubt the cabin crew were glad to see the last of me. Neither my mind nor my eyes would focus properly, but I was aware of being driven along by a silent man in a small electric cart, together with my luggage, medication crate and multi-coloured Mexican leather hat, along shiny corridors, past barriers and queues. A big-time smuggler, I thought dimly, would give his eye teeth for such a smooth entry; or perhaps he would not if it meant feeling the way I did. Then there was Hudie. I recognised him only in outline; my eyes were unable to pick out details. 'Sorry I'm late,' I muttered as he caught me in his arms. 'Sorry about everything, this is not the way I wanted to come home.' I didn't hear what he said, but somehow he got me into the car and we started on the long drive home. I was happy to sit beside him. Beyond that I did not register anything and could not remember a single one of the countless things I had wanted to tell him. Much later he told me that he had recognised me mainly by my clothes, not by my collapsed yellow face, and that he had felt very frightened by my appearance.

At home my mental fog lifted a little and I was delighted to see that Hudie had somehow managed to set up a one-woman version of the Gerson clinic in my large kitchen. The two juice-making machines, the powerful grinder and the simple hydraulic press, stood side by side on the main work surface; the rest of the equipment – vegetable rack, salad shaker, food mill, a variety of graters, bowls and other tools – lay on a trestle table. There were two twenty-eight pound bags of carrots, a crate of apples and several boxes of vegetables, all of them organic, in the glazed-in passage off the kitchen. One of my store cupboards was full of approved foodstuffs: compost grown porridge oats, pure honey, unsulphured prunes, raisins, figs and dates, lentils and mung beans for sprouting, organic English wheat for growing wheatgrass. All this magnificent stuff which Hudie had compiled, with the aid of Margaret Straus's list of essentials, added up to an out-of-season harvest festival. Everything I needed for the therapy was there, everything had been arranged with skill and care, and even in my infernally confused state I felt immense gratitude for the love and intelligence that had gone into all those preparations. I tried to say so, but he shut me up gently and went on explaining the new order in the kitchen and passage, and how the organic produce would be delivered once a week without fail.

Dorothea, my newly recruited assistant who was familiar with the therapy, was not there; she did not work on Saturdays. But she had prepared a generous portion of Hippocrates soup (it smelt exactly the same in London as it had done in Mexico and, presumably, on the island of Cos two thousand five hundred years ago) and also, most importantly for my needs of the moment, a large jugful of enema coffee. I grabbed that jug with the zeal of a junkie reaching for a long-overdue fix. 'Excuse me, darling,' I said to Hudie with some embarrassment, 'I must go upstairs and have an enema at once; it's the only thing that'll make me feel better. I know it sounds weird, but – I can't explain it at the moment.'

He shook his head. 'No need to explain,' he said. 'I've read Dr Gerson's book while you were away, and also Jaquie Davison's, because I wanted to understand

251

what the treatment was all about. So, you see, I know why you feel so rotten and why you need an enema. Or even two. Go ahead and shout if you need anything. You'll find a bottle of purified water in the bathroom, and another eleven out in the passage, so we should be all right for a day or two.'

I crept upstairs, moved and humbled by Hudie's extraordinary kindness, and even by his acceptance of my current situation with all its awkwardness and unlovely needs. He had changed in some way which I was too confused to define. His jovial, easy-going side was still the same, the side that took half-calculated risks and gambles with great good humour and did not mind too much if they did not come off; but now I could sense a new kind of strength in him, a more complete acceptance of things as they were, with no attempt to retouch or avoid them. If our relationship survives the least acceptable parts of the therapy, I thought – the underworld aspects connected with guts and detoxification, sickness and rage – if it survives all that, plus a lengthy withdrawal from normal life, then it will survive anything else, and I will survive, too, if only to make up to him for these bad times.

If I had doubted the instant detoxifying powers of coffee enemas, the next hour would have convinced me for life. Already after the first one I felt astonishingly better; lighter, clearer, with much less pain. The second enema, taken almost immediately afterwards, restored me completely. I was back to normal, except for feeling tired and weak. The storm-lashed stomach, the split skull, the yellow skin and the unfocussable eyes had all righted themselves and I no longer felt feverish or stuck in a painful fog. My vitality began to seep back. Out of sheer relief I now wanted to do everything at once: talk to Hudie, make telephone calls, inspect the garden, open my mail, have a rest, have a bath, unpack, go through the roof with sheer joy at being home again, alive and, if not well, at least much better than I had been at my departure. It was a great cascading moment of almost infinite potential and I was rushing around in my usual chaotic fashion which is as wasteful as it is enjoyable, when Hudie looked at his watch and said, 'Isn't it time you had a juice at last?'

Oh dear. Oh Dr Gerson – forgive me, for I have sinned: I could not even work out how long ago I had had my last juice, and if Hudie had not reminded me, I would have gone on quite happily without one. This dereliction of duty had to stop. I fished out the relevant instruction leaflet from the therapy folder, propped it up behind the machines and sighed. Where did I begin? 'I've watched the maids many times at the clinic,' I said, 'as they were making juices for thirty-odd people at a time, but I've never actually made one myself and I feel very inadequate.'

'Oh come, it can't be all that difficult,' he said. 'Why don't we read the instructions?'

Dorothea, the absent helper, had washed enough apples and carrots for one day's juices. I weighed out eight ounces of each, cut up the apples, topped and tailed the carrots and gingerly put them through the grinder. The powerful American machine uttered a purr and a whine and turned the stuff into rich, moist pulp. Remembering the Mexican maids' procedure, I laid a juicing cloth on a large plate, lined it with a paper towel, piled half the pulp in the middle and wrapped it first in the paper, then in the cloth to make a squelchy little parcel which I then popped in the stainless steel tray of the press. I fastened the screw, inserted the lever, and then worked it up and down, up and down, to make the hydraulic jack exert some of its two-ton pressure, until the juice began to run from the tray into a large glass.

I repeated the process with the remaining pulp. An eight-ounce glass of juice could be pressed in two instalments. The residual pulp in its paper wrap came out of the press as flat and marbled as a linoleum tile. It was hard work and I was not really strong enough for it, but I refused to hand over to Hudie, for it seemed important for me to produce that first portion. Some juice squirted from the tray into my face. 'Excessive zeal,' I snapped at myself. Eventually my first very own self-made juice was glistening in the glass. Then came the medication. I dissolved one jar of mixed potassium salts in two pints of purified water and stirred fast. The Lugol solution was all ready in a small bottle. I added the correct amounts to the juice and drank it, as if my life depended on that glassful. 'The Californian carrots were sweeter and creamier,' I said sadly. We sat at the kitchen table, looking at each other. Making that one juice had taken thirty minutes.

'It'll be much quicker once we've got the hang of it,' said Hudie, guessing my thoughts.

'It had better be,' I replied, 'because each time we also have to dismantle, wash and reassemble two machines, and that means that as soon as one round is completed, we can start on the next one, twelve times a day. Even if we do manage to speed up the process, we'll only have ten or twelve minutes between each round, and I don't think I can cope with that.'

'Ah, hold it, you needn't cope with anything,' he said. 'Dorothea will do all the work and at weekends I'll take over. Don't get yourself into a state. We'll manage. You need your juices and you'll have them.'

I nodded, too depressed to speak. Of course I had realised long ago that doing the therapy at home, even with nearly full-time help, would be much tougher than passively taking it at the clinic, but the horrendously demanding nature of the exercise was only just surfacing into my practical understanding, and it scared me. 'It's going to be quite impossible,' I said at last, 'one thing after another from morning till night, non-stop. And if Dorothea falls ill or walks out, I'll have to do it all – how the hell am I going to cope?'

He put his big, capable hand on mine but did not try

to dismiss my worries. 'We'll cope somehow,' he said, 'because we've no other option. I think we'd better start on another juice, you're in arrears. What comes next on the agenda?'

'A green one. Much more tricky than the carrot and apple one. Where's the leaflet?'

I washed, cut up, weighed and assembled red cabbage, lettuce, watercress, green pepper and apple, and then went through the same procedure as before. This one took even longer to make. My arm was growing tired and I decided to leave the remaining juice-making to Hudie. The red cabbage tinted the juice a glorious shade of purple. 'So that's what you call a *green* juice,' said Hudie, preparing to wash up the machines. He applied the same dash and thoroughness to washing up as to everything else he did. The juice, both sweet and tart, tasted comforting. As I watched him being efficient at the sink, I had to laugh at the absurdity of the situation.

'My poor love,' I said, 'you're so incredibly good about this whole business, although red roses and good wine would be more your style than cabbage stalks and carrot juice. I've no idea what we've done to deserve this development, but there it is, and thank you for not running away.'

'Don't be silly. Why should I run away now that you're back? I only felt tempted once or twice to pack it in and clear out while you were away and I couldn't even get you on the phone – all I got was the Mexican operator complaining about their useless system. That's when I got really frustrated. But now no one's going to run away from here until you've finished your treatment. After that I suppose we'll run away together. Now look, why don't you have a rest before we start on the liver juice? I imagine that'll be the worst job of all.'

I did not feel like resting and made some telephone calls instead. My mother, whose tears of joy and grief are always close to the surface, cried a great deal while

255

I tried to talk to her, but eventually she calmed down. Her main concern was to know that I was back in safe, familiar London. Catherine and John gave me a rousing welcome and arranged to drop in on the following day. I dialled a few more numbers. It was like returning from the dead to be able to say 'I'm back!' and almost hear the tiny imaginary clicks of being reconnected with my friends.

Back in the kitchen we tried and nearly failed to make a liver-cum-carrot juice. Despite our joint efforts and the dreadful bloody mess they resulted in, the extra-young calves' liver Hudie had obtained through a local butcher (it was of the kind normally bought up by pharmaceutical firms, being too tasteless to eat) yielded very little juice, barely one-third of the tumblerful I had drunk three times a day in Mexico. Hudie blamed my inefficient electric mincer, I blamed the liver, and told him about the near-mutiny at the clinic when the liver supply from Florida had broken down for a whole day, driving several patients frantic with worry. 'It's nothing to do with what you're taught about the therapy,' I explained. 'You brainwash yourself into thinking that, say, the liver juice is your main defence and main tool of recovery, you turn it into a kind of magical talisman, so that if for some reason you can't have it for a day or two, your confidence collapses and you fear the worst. I don't want to get like that, but the temptation is there.'

Washing up after the liver exercise was a long, sticky job which Hudie insisted on doing. I wandered around, trying to prepare a meal, trying to remember all the things that needed doing, but the longer the list grew, the more I panicked. Cook, eat, wash up, make three more juices, have two more enemas, soak seeds for sprouting, make two pints of coffee concentrate for tomorrow, wash and boil the juicing cloths – the tasks seemed too numerous to be carried out by any ordinary mortal. But then my panic subsided and I thought it was marvellous that I was worrying myself silly about the demands and details of the therapy but not at all about my disease, as if I took my recovery for granted.

'You see? We've done everything. Even your stewed fruit is ready for breakfast,' Hudie said two hours later, surveying the once more tidy kitchen with the air of a victorious Roman general. The plural was complimentary: he had done almost all the work. 'Now you can go and sleep off your jet lag; frankly I'm surprised to see you still upright. Stay in bed as long as you like, I'll make the juices tomorrow.' The man was a miracle, still calm and cheerful after such an endless, thorny day.

'I don't deserve you,' I said and went straight to bed.

Now it was the Thames at the bottom of the road, not the Pacific, and instead of being surrounded by fellow Gersonites I was all alone, tête-à-tête with the therapy, embarking on what Dr Hesse had called an epic enterprise. It felt epic all right, frighteningly so. I lay in the dark, contemplating the prospect of sixteen months of tough, solitary dedication to the therapy, to the exclusion of all else. It felt like taking vows and entering an enclosed order where I was to be the only nun, both pledged to obedience and also put in charge of the rules. That was crazy enough, undertaking to tackle a major life-threatening disease at home, on a do-it-yourself basis, with only rudimentary marginal help. But below the surface, on the non-physical level, I could sense another strange process at work which felt just as important as the complexities of the therapy.

What was it about? I spent some time trying to grasp and define the process, but when the mental approach failed, I reverted to the old technique of trying to get an image for the elusive sensation. What came up promptly was a very large funnel. Its wide top was brightly lit against a beautiful, dreamy landscape, but down below its narrow end led into a pool of darkness. While watching the funnel inside my closed eyelids I had the sensation of being somewhere halfway down its body, just above the point where it narrowed into a tube. Well yes, absolutely correct, I thought; when thinking fails, you can always trust your images. I now saw that the baffling inner process I was trying to grasp was funnel-shaped indeed and that it was forcing me into even smaller spaces. The first phase of my illness had banished me from the boundless, carefree arena of the strong and healthy, from the bright, sunlit scenery at the top, into a less assured, more circumscribed existence. The second phase, corresponding to the narrowing of the funnel, had removed me altogether from my world and landed me in the strict microcosm of the clinic; yet even there I had enjoyed companionship, study and new experiences. But now I was being forced into the long final descent through the tube of the funnel into sixteen months of solitary confinement at home, imprisoned in a dawn-to-dusk routine with very little leisure and space, minimal company, and the solitude of travelling alone.

It seemed like a non-physical death, being cornered, stripped and pushed into such a tiny, lonely place, exiled from the ordinary world, reduced to my own resources, and I did not much like the thick blackness at the bottom. But then, I thought, I have chosen the trip, I might just as well proceed in an orderly fashion and find out where it takes me.

Just before I dropped off to sleep, my memory presented me with a half-forgotten story, used in Buddhist meditation, which I had once loved. It is about an Indian prince who gave a ring to his jeweller and asked him to engrave on it a sentence that would sustain him in adversity and restrain him in times of success. In due course the jeweller returned the ring, engraved with three words: 'It will pass.'

15

SOMEHOW, BY THE skin of our teeth Hudie and I got through that first weekend without skipping a single part of the therapy or snapping at each other out of sheer exasperation over the endless monotonous chores. Once again he did most of the work; I was still weary after my dreadful journey. But I got my second wind after dinner when Catherine and John arrived, loaded with spring flowers and, in John's case, enough joyful energy to set the place dancing. We did in fact dance around in a rapturous reunion polka, and when at last we sat down, Catherine held my hand for a while, as if there had been some risk of my dematerialising and vanishing into a large, remote container labelled 'Mexico'. There was so much to say to them that I gave up and just sat there in unaccustomed silence, beaming with contentment. It felt reassuring to be surrounded by my closest friends and allies at another milestone along my cancer pilgrimage and to hear their voices instead of just reading their letters.

'You're thin,' Catherine said later when we went upstairs for a spell of woman-talk and for her to inspect my self-restoring skin graft.

'I'm seven pounds lighter than when you last saw me.'

'I don't mean just that; on your diet I'd expect you to be underweight. But you're also thin in substance, as if your atomic density had dropped. You look rather ethereal, in fact.'

'Ethereal? How marvellous – nobody's ever called me

that! I feel quite normal, whatever that means, so you'll have to monitor me and tell me how I'm doing from your point of view.'

'I'll do that gladly,' Catherine said, 'but I hope there are other, more reliable ways to check your progress?'

'Not really. Except blood and urine tests, and those don't tell you all that much. Personally I think I'll use my leg as my healing barometer. As long as it keeps growing back, there's nothing to worry about, because if my various systems weren't on the mend, there could be no reconstruction going on. You've no idea what it feels like to know that my poor battered leg has started rebuilding itself. It's awesome and also very funny, the nearest thing to a lizard regrowing its tail. I'd like to know how the body does it. How does it know, for instance, just how much flesh to grow and when to stop in order to get the shape right. Do you realise, that's the exact opposite of what cancer cells do. They don't know when to stop, which is cell madness. What my leg is doing seems to be cell wisdom.'

'Well, well. I've known a few wise heads in this life, but yours is the first wise leg I've met,' Catherine said, contemplating my maverick limb. Even in the few days since I had first noticed the reconstruction process, the new flesh underneath the skin graft had grown thicker and sturdier. 'All I can do is to bow to your miraculous hind leg,' she said eventually. 'You're probably walking on a piece of medical history. For goodness' sake look after it, don't fall under a bus. Once you've grown back a large chunk, we'll organise busloads of people to come and admire your leg and perhaps even touch it. You'll have to charge an entrance fee, of course.'

'Like in a stately home? What a good idea. By the time I finish with this fiendishly expensive therapy, I'll probably go around with a begging bowl. A miraculous hind leg might be a useful source of income.'

'I daresay you'll find some other source, too, when the time is ripe,' Catherine said evenly. Over the years, having witnessed each other's financial ups and downs and apparently insoluble crises, we had reached the conclusion that one's true needs are always met, often in hilariously unexpected ways, so that worrying about them is a waste of time. 'But tell me, apart from your leg and your finances, what does it feel like to be you just now?'

I pondered that for a while. 'I feel embattled. Besieged by practical chores, wrapped up in the therapy, almost confined to it, as if it were a cell. I know what I'm doing and why I'm doing it, but I've no overview and no particular awareness of myself as I exist beyond the therapy. The inner dimension is still missing. Seeing you and John again makes me realise how far I've drifted from it. Last night it struck me how both my inner and my outer space were getting smaller and smaller . . . it's like being a plant that's forced back into the seed it's grown from. Does that make sense?'

'It does to me, although I don't know how a botanist might react. Going back to the seed stage sounds a good way towards regeneration; you can't get much more basic than that. Oh, my friend, trust you to get recycled without all that tiresome business of having to die down, get composted and re-sown! You've always claimed to be an eccentric gardener and now you're proving it. I shouldn't worry too much about having no overview at the moment.'

'But I don't like being exiled into this total body-world!'

'You're not. Come on, you know this as well as I do – the inner process does go on, even if you're not aware of it for a while. It might be a good idea to trust the process and more or less forget about it.'

'Oh, very well, as long as you occasionally ask me what it feels like to be me. Otherwise I'll just drift.'

'I doubt that. But of course I'll ask you again. And again.'

We went downstairs and rejoined the men. 'Do you

mind us drinking Scotch,' John asked, 'when all you get is carrot juice?' No, I did not, I had no wish to drink, and when Catherine invited me to sniff her glass, I found the once loved smell of Scotch unpleasantly harsh, no more alluring than dry-cleaning fluid.

'God, I shan't have any vices left by the time I get well,' I complained. 'I'll be plain healthy and boring . . . who'll want to know a non-smoking, teetotal vegetarian? Are there any worthwhile vices that don't clash with the therapy?' A few interesting suggestions were made and the conversation was still in full spate when John and Catherine rose to go. I protested in vain.

'It's probably long past your bedtime,' they said, and for a moment the indignant child in me saw them as a pair of dear, concerned adults, about to disappear into the wider world where I could not follow them.

That first carefully timed visit set the pattern of my social life for a long time to come. I was forced to accept that the cast-iron timetable of the therapy and the care and maintenance of my fluctuating energy had to take precedence over all else. Friends' visits and even telephone calls had to be fitted in between enemas and other chores. Later, when Hudie began to take me out for brief drives on Sunday mornings, our outings were limited by the fact that the single carrot and apple juice which I was allowed to take along in a thermos flask had to be drunk within two hours of being made, and that the one to follow had to be freshly made in time and on time. This was worse than being Cinderella; she only had to watch out for the stroke of midnight, while I had a juice deadline (all right, lifeline) every sixty minutes. During the early phase of the regime, as my frustration built up, I sometimes saw my daily routine as a subtle but sadistic punishment worthy of the milder regions of some modern Inferno, the endless torture of being assaulted by juices at one end and enemas at the other, interrupting all else, in a setting of apparent ease and comfort. But these exaggerated fantasies were rare and ceased altogether when I was allowed to cut my five daily enemas to four and, several months later, to three. After the total bondage of the super-intensive therapy every cut, every reduction in chores felt like liberation.

But is it really necessary to observe the programme so strictly, friends kept asking in the following weeks and months; was not this every-hour-on-the-hour juice routine exaggerated, too Teutonic in its precision and generally overdone? What would happen, they asked, if just for once you rebelled and drank only six juices, not thirteen, and went to the theatre instead? Would not the change do you more good than the juices? Those were perfectly reasonable questions, but I honestly did not know the answers. Having committed myself to the treatment, I was determined to stick to it without changes or short cuts, because that was the only way to see if it worked for me. Anyway, it was not part of a guinea-pig's brief to redesign the experiment it was participating in. And beyond the guinea-pig level, as a patient wanting to recover, I would not have dared to bend the rules. Charlotte's cautionary case histories of negligent or rule-breaking patients had made a deep impression on me.

On the first Monday after my return home, Dorothea, the trained helper, arrived with a bounce and a flourish. She was a tall, strong young woman, rather plain, with the vague smile and uncertain glance of the extremely short sighted. I welcomed her warmly and would have done so even if she had been four feet tall and bald, with purple eyes; by then I knew that without outside help the therapy would soon collapse around my ears. Dorothea was a much-travelled girl from the North of England, deeply 'into' alternative medicine. She had attended one of Margaret Straus's seminars, read The Book and worked briefly with a Gerson patient. Above all, she was enthusiastic about the therapy and seemed ideal for the job, so that I handed her the reins of the kitchen with relief. I knew there would be problems. In a letter from Baltimore my dear, much-missed Becky had hinted at the awkwardness of having a stranger in charge of one's household. In her case it was a series of strangers provided by the local Church; nice, kind ladies, according to Becky, (but then would she have been uncomplimentary about anyone this side of Satan?) who were nevertheless 'a disturbing influence'. Dorothea, I guessed, would not be trouble-free either, but I was glad to have her around from nine to five, Monday to Friday, until further notice.

She was a fast and energetic worker. She was also astoundingly messy, scattering liquid and solid debris in all directions and, despite her very strong glasses, not noticing the sticky trail that built up behind her as she rushed around the kitchen. Never mind, I thought, contemplating the rapid deterioration of the décor, she is producing meals and juices on time, she is pleasant if somewhat overpowering. I really must not worry about sticky surfaces and glasses cloudy with fingerprints, must not mind if she lets the enema coffee overboil and flood the cooker or if she forgets to remove the burnt bits from the soup casserole.

Hudie, himself a fussy perfectionist, sensed my misgivings and did his best to dispel them. 'Try to ignore it, darling,' he insisted when I complained about Dorothea's slapdash habits. 'We'll redecorate the kitchen when the therapy is over. Those beetroot stains on the wall will fade, and the marks on the floor aren't too bad. All that matters is that the girl keeps the juicer going. You mustn't mind the rest.'

Yes, quite. But deep down I did mind. And it puzzled and amused me that having achieved detachment in the most important areas of life, including my own survival or death, I was now unable to muster any when it came to the state of my kitchen floor. Clearly, the old, familiar gap between theory and practice was as wide as ever.

Soon after Dorothea's arrival Hudie drove me to Dr

Montague's surgery for a general examination and check-up. As I entered his consulting room, I felt like a pilgrim returning to home base, bearing tales of remote lands, and in fact Dr Montague wanted to know all about my experience at the clinic before taking a good look at me. 'One day perhaps I'll visit the Gerson clinic and see it for myself,' he said with a shy little smile. He was as quiet and subdued as ever and only became more animated at the sight of my re-fleshing leg. 'That's most unusual,' he murmured, gently touching the freshly regrown part. 'I hope you have a "before" picture of your leg?' Well yes, I said, a picture existed and I would try to get a print of it; what I longed to know was just how much of the mutilated part was likely to regrow in the long run. Impossible to tell, he said and moved on to examine the tumour. Yes, it had grown bigger since January, but as it had also risen towards the surface, he could not assess just how much it had grown. His cool, matter of fact reaction to the greatly increased lump was reassuring. So was the fact that he found no other lumps, however long he searched for them. My general condition, he said, seemed satisfactory, and he only hoped that I would be able to persevere with the therapy.

In the course of subsequent visits I realised that if Dr Montague called my condition satisfactory, then I was doing remarkably well indeed; he was not given to hyperbole. But behind his reserve there was a depth of caring and kindness, and during my endless months of battling on with the therapy it comforted me to know that Dr Montague was around and accessible.

Next to him my other main support was Margaret Straus. During my first few confused weeks at home I rang her whenever I ran into a problem to which there was no answer either in The Book or in the lecture notes I had taken at the clinic. Margaret's answers were always crisp and to the point, and in matters of therapy she was as uncompromising as her mother, Charlotte

Gerson. Their strictness was meant to protect both the patient and the reputation of the therapy; their worst fear was that people might take up the Gerson programme, bend and relax its rules to suit their convenience and then when, predictably, it did not work, dismiss it as worthless.

A few weeks after my return from Mexico my awareness of time changed drastically. The way I experienced it, time had become faceless and undifferentiated. It rolled along like an endless sausage, day following day with no distinguishing marks to break up the monotony. The pattern did not change. I was busy with therapy chores from 7am to Dorothea's arrival at nine, and again from her departure at five until eight-thirty or nine in the evening, the length of my last shift depending on the amount of cleaning up I had to do after her. While she was around I could read, write, enjoy friends' visits, rest, always subject to interruptions; I also had to take an hour's exercise a day in whatever form. The whole business smacked of an invalid's version of galley-slavery. I could only bear it by living from one day to the next and keeping a modest horizon. The repetitive routine acted like a sedative, mild enough to let me function yet blotting out all the sheen and flavour of being.

My concept of space had also changed. Being reduced to very short walks in the immediate neighbourhood and forced into close contact with the vegetable kingdom, I became a connoisseur of tiny areas and fine detail. I got to know personally every duck and Canada goose on the Thames and every crack in the towpath alongside it. I learnt to read the messages conveyed by neighbours' curtain materials and studied the condition of their front gardens, including their choice of fencing. And on weekend mornings, washing mounds of vegetables at the sink, I often felt empathy with the produce I was handling. I seemed to experience the essence of each beetroot, potato and celery stalk that passed through my hands; the perfect co-ordination of qualities that added up to a spring onion – shape, colour, smell, flavour, texture essentially right. I had to admit that a passionate extrovert like myself needed the close confinement of my current lifestyle to discover the essence of humble things, and it was thrilling to become fully aware of the marvellous structure and regal glow of a red cabbage leaf. But, like all mystical experiences, such moments also faded, and much of the time I just felt like a plain cabbage myself.

My most vivid dream in those early weeks concerned Mr Lennox. In the dream I sat opposite him in his consulting room, stark naked but unembarrassed: it was the kind of dream nakedness that symbolises total openness, with nothing to hide. I wanted to show him the new flesh on my leg and tell him about the Gerson therapy, but he refused to look or listen and kept chanting, 'We're going to chop! We're going to chop!' To my surprise – for such abandoned behaviour was out of character for him – he even drummed on the table to the beat of his chant. When I saw that I was getting nowhere, I said sharply, 'We're *not* going to chop!' and walked out. He followed me, smiling and chatting, right down to Oxford Street where he stopped me outside the long-vanished Marshall and Snelgrove department store, a place I only remember for its faded olde worlde atmosphere.

'Please come in and have a look at my new premises,' he said. 'They'll be rather nice once the workmen finish the job.' As we stepped inside, I saw that the whole ground floor had been turned into a luxurious waiting room, complete with chandeliers and reproduction furniture. There were workmen and ladders everywhere. 'The trouble is,' Mr Lennox explained, 'that the builders are quite unable to get the stairs into position. I've no idea why, and everything's held up.' Indeed, an elegant wooden staircase stood in the middle of the vast hall, ready to be installed, except that it had nowhere to go;

it had not occurred to anyone to make a suitable opening in the grey concrete ceiling above.

'But this is ridiculous,' I said to Mr Lennox. 'Can't you see what's wrong? It's not enough to buy the staircase and the stair carpet, you also have to gain access to the next level. At this rate you'll never get beyond the ground floor.' And there the dream ended.

I did not know whether my dream was a fair assessment of how Mr Lennox might respond if I visited him – fully dressed, of course – in real life. But remembering the authoritative way in which he had told me that diet had nothing to do with cancer, I did not think he would change his views on my say-so or concede that chopping out tumours was no long-term answer to cancer. In that light it seemed accurate to see him as being stuck on the ground floor, unable to reach a higher, more holistic understanding of disease. All right, I was not objective, for I still felt angry with him for having uselessly slaughtered my leg, and my resentment had obviously coloured the dream. But even so I did not think it was too far out.

So far, so unfair? Perhaps. Yet there was also a deeper level of interpretation, the one on which all the *dramatis personae* of the dream represent unconscious aspects of ourselves. Come on, face it, I said to myself: in some way I, too, am stuck on the ground floor, although I have plenty of stairs and ladders to take me higher up, but I am not using them. I am doggedly, devotedly pursuing the therapy in all its material details but not doing anything else to promote healing. I am not working on my buried emotions or tackling unfinished business from the past. Worst of all, I am not trying to identify the psychological factors that might have contributed to my disease.

There was no getting away from it: without inner work the Gerson therapy was just as one-sided in its body-centredness as the orthodox treatments. I knew of only one reference in The Book that pointed beyond the purely physical: 'It should be remembered that a successful therapy requires harmony of the physical and psychological functions, in order to achieve a restoration of the body in its entirety.' True, but not enough. Perhaps there was no need for further emphasis on the psychological side in Dr Gerson's lifetime, for he must have had the true physician-healer's charisma that awakens and aligns the patient's total self without pep talks or didactic explanations; but that non-transferable, non-verbal gift had died with him, and nothing had come to take its place. Unless I provided the missing dimension, I would remain as stuck on the ground floor of my 'new premises' as Mr Lennox was on his.

Déjà vu, déjà dit? Yes, of course. I had a similar moment of insight at La Mesa and a similar urge to deepen the healing experience. But nothing happened, because Lily and Tom invaded my space and drove me berserk instead. All right, let me try again. See what happens this time.

What happened this time was that barely had I started on a modest programme of relaxation and meditation when Dorothea began to play up, making me increasingly uncomfortable. She still did her job well, but her mess-making was growing barely tolerable, and so was her bossiness. If I picked up a sponge to wipe a sticky surface or tried to sort out a jumble of cutlery, she swooped on me with loud reproaches, as if I had been a trespasser in my own kitchen. Our conflict worked on several levels. Her carelessness triggered off in me the obsessionally clean housewife whom I much preferred dormant if not dead, while her bossiness awakened my primitive territorial instincts. She was on a power trip, but in my weak state I was not able to put her in her place. Besides, in the shadow of her mood swings, I feared that if I voiced any objection, she might storm out and leave me high and dry.

Yet we also had good days when she would be sunny, charming, thoughtful and great fun. But more often than not she would arrive bad-tempered and taciturn and stay like that all day. Her love life was in poor shape, she told me, adding that whenever the blood of her Macedonian grandmother bubbled up in her veins, she flew off the handle and could not control her moods. Unfortunately, her exotic granny's genes were pretty active in those days, sweeping aside the more stable genes of her North Country ancestors, and I picked up a lot of repressed violence behind Dorothea's conduct.

The exact state of her eyesight also puzzled me. Judging by the condition of my kitchen, her sight was about as good as that of the proverbial bat, but as I could not be sure, I gave her the benefit of the doubt. Things came to a crunch in early May, when my weekly shipment of fresh young lettuces, used in the green juices, arrived full of fresh young slugs, a dozen or more per lettuce. Over the weekend I removed large numbers, flushing them down the sink. It was the price one paid for using chemical-free, organic produce. Not until the following Tuesday did I remember the creatures, which is when I said to Dorothea, 'Those slugs in last week's lettuces are a nuisance – you must be sick and tired of them by now.' She looked astonished. 'Slugs? What slugs?' she asked. 'I haven't noticed any. What do they look like?'

My stomach rocked. I took a lettuce from the refrigerator, removed its polythene cloak and pulled the leaves apart. Sure enough, the slugs, now rather chilled, were neatly tucked up inside. 'Here – can't you see them?' I asked.

Dorothea peered uncertainly at the lettuce. 'Oh, those?' she asked in a voice that was a tacit admission in itself. No more was said. I went upstairs and lay down, feeling sick. My only consolation was that if slugs had indeed formed part of my green juices over two days, at least they were strictly organic.

But then, as more and more things went wrong and I

considered the number of garden pests that might glide unseen into my food and drink, I realised the need for action. I advertised locally and when a suitable girl appeared, I gave notice to Dorothea. She did not seem surprised or ask why I was dismissing her. Perhaps she had been expecting the sack. But at our final goodbye she dropped her mask of let's-see-how-far-I-can-go arrogance and looked sad and bewildered. I wondered if I should talk to her and try to explain. But she walked out and I never saw her again.

That was how the tragi-comical soap opera of my helpers began. Apart from Dorothea I employed a total of five over sixteen months. All were young girls aged between sixteen and twenty-two, but that was the only thing they had in common, for one was marvellous, one was good, but three were so awful that at times I almost agreed with the patient back in Mexico who had once declared that the helpers were a worse problem than the cancer. Well, no, not quite, but pretty damned close on the whole, because the trivial, petty worries caused by inadequate helpers made my daily life even pettier and more detail-ridden.

The one and only marvellous girl, Harriet, who took over from Dorothea, stayed on for three months and spoilt me for the rest of the therapy, for she was both an excellent worker and good company. She learned the routine quickly; she was bright, amusing and full of vitality. Moreover, she knew and liked fresh vegetables, unlike most of the other girls who had been reared on tinned junk, and did not know a leek from a swede and had never seen a green pepper or fresh garden peas. They were addicted to crisps, peanuts and dreadful sweets and obviously thought my diet completely crazy. The most useless girl of all, Cindy, smothered her freshly prepared organic lunches with tomato ketchup or salad cream which she had asked me to provide; she could not understand how any household survived without those two items.

271

Cindy was good-natured, placid and unteachable. Once, when she had made the same stupid mistake for the sixth time and I asked her whether she ever listened to me, she broke into a radiant smile and said, 'Oh yes, I do, but what you say goes in one ear and out the other.' Cindy existed in a haze of pop music, cigarettes (which she smoked in the garden) and sensational stories from the more lurid tabloids. Without those stimuli she promptly sank into zombiehood.

She did not last long. Nor did Pauline, a part-time model with a sexy wiggle, who burst into tears on her fifth working day and sobbed noisily. The job was too lonely and my house was too quiet, she wailed, she simply could not bear it. Considering that her previous job had been in a jeans boutique in Oxford Street, her distress was understandable. So was mine. I had barely managed to teach her the routine when she already asked to be released.

Then came Moira, a dark, brooding drop-out from a North London commune. Moira was 'into' countless esoteric theories and techniques without really understanding any of them, but this did not stop her from preaching at me out of her profound ignorance. Moira was relentlessly earnest and humourless, a potential beauty heavily disguised under bunchy garments in puce and violet, colours which she told me had the most powerful wisdom vibes. The only vibes I could sense conveyed an urgent need for laundering. Moira was an unhappy girl, an archetypal rebel without cause, direction or structure. She was obviously struggling to find her identity, but the half-baked ideas which she kept picking up in the phoney Himalayas of West Kilburn confused her even more. I was aware of her needfulness and at times we had long talks which seemed to help her a little. But on each occasion after a few days of peace and friendly co-existence Moira would turn bolshie again and treat me with scorn and hostility. I realised that she was projecting onto me all the negative authority figures she had ever known and, knowing her family history, I sympathised with her conflicts, until Hudie reminded me that it was Moira's job to look after my physical needs, not mine to give her psychotherapy.

Moira's gloomy reign in my kitchen ended dramatically when she stuck a vegetable knife into the powerful American grinder which was working at full speed; later she claimed that she had wanted to shift a piece of beetroot that had got stuck. She stopped the motor immediately, but the long blade had already wound itself around the cutter inside the steel housing and could not be removed. When I entered the kitchen, I was shocked to see the melodramatic sight of the black knife handle sticking out from the top of the grinder. It looked as if my precious machine, the king-pin of the juice therapy, had been stabbed through the heart by Moira. I tried to pull out the knife, but it remained firmly jammed inside the murdered grinder.

I got into a terrible state which was barely short of hysteria, for I was terrified of having to interrupt the therapy for any length of time. But Moira was unrepentant. 'Perhaps this is a sign that you should come off the therapy and try something else,' she said in her ponderous high-priestess voice. 'You've got to read the signs and go with the flow.'

I subdued a strong urge to hit her. 'Be quiet,' I shouted, 'I've had enough of your pretentious rubbish – don't make things worse, they're bad enough as it is.' She tried once more to present herself as an instrument of destiny, but I silenced her with one look. Eventually, to my deep relief, my kind and highly skilled neighbour managed to tease the ruined knife out of the mercifully undamaged grinder. The next day I took urgent steps to replace Moira.

My last helper, Colleen, stayed nearly to the end of my eighteen-month stint. Except for her regrettable habit of taking days off and offering the most unlikely excuses for her frequent absences, she was as good as gold; a sturdy, tough, lovable little sparrow of not quite seventeen, already battered by life and accordingly programmed for disappointment and failure. Colleen was clean, neat, thorough and – when she did turn up for work – utterly reliable, enabling me to spend much of the day free from chores and worries. When she did not turn up – always ringing at the last moment with some fanciful alibi – I had to buckle down to the job myself. It was just as well that these episodes occurred during the last phase of the intensive therapy when I had enough strength and energy to do all the chores myself and not drop with fatigue until the evening.

But in the early phase, in the spring of 1981, I would have found it hard to imagine ever having that kind of energy again. My low-protein diet just about allowed me to tick over but left no margin for any extra effort. Once, when the liver supply broke down for nearly two weeks, I suffered nasty fits of faintness, like the heroines of Victorian romances. But on the whole I was feeling well, free of pain, waiting for more flare-ups (having had none since my dreadful flight home), and ticking off every week in my diary to mark the achievement of having survived another seven days.

One fine spring day, when my dwarf apple trees were just about to burst into blossom, I received a letter from Becky with a Californian postmark instead of the usual Baltimore one. 'I know that this will come as a shock to you,' she wrote. 'I have returned to La Gloria six weeks after having tried the therapy at home. I developed an infection that needed big-gun antibiotics. This in turn created a need to suspend all medication on the therapy. I got in touch with Dr Arturo and he suggested I return to be stabilised.' Her handwriting looked faint and uneven. My heart grew heavier with every line I read. 'The flight here was horrendous. I've been here two weeks, am confined to bed, and am fighting an uphill battle. They took an X-ray of my lungs

274

and now they are waiting for the previous X-ray from home, so they can compare the rate of growth and decide what to do.' I read on, with tears rolling down my face, although I was not crying; it was as if I had been hearing Becky's soft, eternally apologetic voice through a thick curtain. 'But I'm so happy that by and large the therapy is working for you,' the letter ended. 'Anyway, my love, carry on the good fight. God be with you.'

I immediately wrote to her at the clinic, begging for news, however brief, but somehow I knew that none would come. That odd, poignant moment at La Gloria way back in January, when I knew with awful certainty that one of us, Becky or I, would not recover, now shifted into position. Everything I knew about her had signalled right from the beginning that she was too nice, too self-effacing and gentle to fight for her life, but even so I had hoped that under duress she would change sufficiently to reverse or at least halt her disease. Well, I had been wrong and I felt infinitely sad. After Dorothea's departure I lit the large blue candle that John and Catherine had brought back for me from Rocamadour, the ancient French sanctuary of a Black Madonna, and sat quietly, thinking of Becky.

I did not hear from her again. Some time later, in response to my query, Charlotte wrote and confirmed that Becky had gone home from the clinic in a very bad condition and was probably no longer alive. But by the time that news arrived I had already done my mourning.

Shortly afterwards I had a telephone call from Karen, the young girl who had looked more dead than alive when I had first met her at La Gloria. She was back in London, feeling much better, and finding the therapy difficult to run at home. We talked at length, comparing notes and swapping practical hints. I was overjoyed to hear her sounding almost perky. Neither of us could visit the other – we lived at opposite ends of London – but we agreed to keep in touch on the telephone.

I lit my blue candle once more, this time for joy. At that moment I seemed to exist at a level of experience where a primitive gesture, such as lighting a candle, can have several meanings.

16

I CANNOT GIVE a proper account of how I got through the final phase of the intensive therapy. The truth is that I hardly know myself. All I know is that it was a kind of desert crossing, a long, slow trek through the wilderness, with only a few landmarks to guide me, but blessed with a sprinkling of oases that grew brighter as time went on. All the things that I most disliked – confinement, monotony, isolation, enforced passivity – closed in and became part of my daily routine, so much so that even complaining about them would have been predictable and therefore pointless.

Eventually I came to accept them. All right, so this was to be a period of dullness and incarceration, of body centredness and lack of stimulus, and no amount of protest and indignation would change that; perhaps it was best to get on with it and see the process as an extraordinary and highly irregular training course in the art of acceptance. Having studied Oriental philosophies for years, I now had the chance, or rather the unavoidable task of putting them into practice. So I tried and failed and tried again and again to practise glad acceptance and get a true view of reality while marching ahead with the remorseless routine of diet, juices, enemas, medication, castor oil, injections, exercise, good days, bad days, flare-ups, fits of anxiety and panic, bouts of apprehension, wondering and doubting; but at a deeper level I frequently caught a different note that allowed me to transcend the all too tangible side of existence for a moment or two and also signalled that I was moving in the right direction. It was an indescribable note; for a long time I was unable to put words to it, until at last what came up as the nearest verbal approximation was a haunting line from the Upanishads, 'O my soul, remember past strivings, remember! O my soul, remember past strivings, remember!' It was an odd message to arrive into a reality so closely circumscribed by piles of muddy carrots and a deep sense of exile, but it felt right and I accepted it with joy.

The daily routine was often disrupted by practical difficulties. But whether it was the juice press that broke down or my helper who needed a lift from halfway across London during a transport strike, Hudie always stepped in like a jovial guardian angel and sorted things out. He took on everything and solved all my practical problems. Nothing was too much, nothing ruffled his optimism, cheerfulness and dedicated caring; not even my spells of unreasonable behaviour. 'Why don't you ever lose your temper with me?' I asked him one day when even I could not bear my nasty, irritable, childish self any longer. 'If you go on repressing all the negative stuff, it'll blow up when we're least able to handle it. I'd rather you weren't so unflappable!'

But he shrugged off my qualms. 'The way you live now,' he said, 'you've every right to get impatient and awkward every now and then. I'll snap at you when you're well again.' And, with his generous heart, he left it at that.

There were small pleasures, such as my first portion of de-fatted cottage cheese and saltless sourdough bread, authorised by Charlotte in the sixth month of the therapy. Both tasted indescribably delicious, food fit for angels. Sometimes I obtained a bunch of unsprayed grapes or an organically grown melon, and these rare treats awakened my taste buds until the next baked turnip put them into a coma again. The forbidden foods and drinks, which I kept for visitors, only bothered me occasionally. Accessible but taboo, they made me appreciate what a eunuch might have felt in a harem. Only once in sixteen months did I feel strongly tempted to chuck in the therapy, shake off all chains and restrictions and, as a symbol of insurgence, go out and eat a sumptuous Indian meal even if it killed me (which it probably would have done). Having spun the fantasy that far, I found that the sweet remembered flavours of fine curries and chutneys stirred me on an emotional level which added fuel to the temptation. The same night my unconscious sent me a strong reprimand in the form of a dream which showed me my zodiacal symbol, the scorpion, clinging to a rock in a storm. It was a small brown creature, lashed mercilessly by wind and rain, but it hung on, looking as indestructible as the rock, indifferent to the storm. Point taken, I thought. That puny, unheroic image pulled me up more sharply than the vision of a shining warrior might have done.

My body was steadily restoring itself. After six months the right side of the huge excision on my right leg had regrown completely. On the more devastated left side progress was slower. Other parts of my body also showed signs of repairing old injuries, just as Charlotte had predicted. In every instance the old problem grew worse, sometimes alarmingly so, before clearing up for good. And so, one by one, my faulty parts joined this great round of spring cleaning: my left eye, always the weaker of the two, my incompletely healed rib broken five years before, my right knee injured in adolescence, all went haywire in their different ways before healing completely.

Two small instances in that chain of self-healing were of a cosmetic nature. My greying, fading eyebrows turned dark again, while the large brown spot on my jaw which Dr Colville, the dermatologist, had called an irremovable age spot, simply disappeared. Those tiny signs of rejuvenation pleased me greatly; not just for reasons of vanity but also because, taken together with the more important repair jobs, they proved that the body could restore itself in the second half of middle age when conventional wisdom would expect it to accelerate into irreversible decline. But then did anyone know just what feats of self-healing the body was capable of under ideal conditions?

Contemplating the ideal conditions created by my diabolical regime, I worked out that in sixteen months I would consume a total of six thousand two hundred and forty juices, equalling one hundred and sixty-two gallons. I also decided that on the Gerson therapy it was meaningless to think in terms of the carrot and the stick; in our case the carrot was the stick.

Flare-ups were the only unpredictable factor in my clockwork existence. I never knew when the next one would hit me. Each one started with deep fatigue and unnatural hunger and continued with nausea, a splitting headache, niggly pains and alarming weakness. The worst ones also brought on fits of vomiting. Morning sickness without pregnancy and a vile hangover without the preliminary pleasures of alcohol was one way to describe the experience, yet thanks to my training at La Gloria I was able to feel glad – well, moderately glad at least – whenever a flare-up felled me, for it showed that I was detoxifying fast.

I survived a total of twenty-six flare-ups during that period. Some of the worst hit me on weekday evenings when I was alone in the house. At first I found this depressing, but later got quite used to flaring in solitude. Once or twice I reread the chapter on flare-ups in The Book to make sure that my symptoms tallied with those on the official list. Later I hit on the idea of listening to one of Charlotte's tapes, and her clear, no-nonsense voice reassured me at once. It also reminded me of the many times in Mexico when I had asked her petulantly why I was not producing flare-ups. 'Okay, now you've got one,' I imagined her saying with her bright, blue-eyed smile, 'get on with it.' Quite right, Charlotte, I thought, as the tape rolled on.

Most of my flare-ups lasted for twenty-four hours or less. In between them I was feeling increasingly well and strong. My weight was back at its normal level and Catherine declared that I no longer struck her as ethereal. In fact, I now looked healthier than some of my visitors who arrived looking pale, tired, with lack-lustre eyes, so that more and more it was I who felt concerned about my friends' health instead of the other way round.

The worst part of the desert crossing was that I still had to cope with periods of boiling anger; nothing as violent as my ten-day rage at La Mesa, but pretty explosive nonetheless. Once again I recognised these fits of spluttering, muttering, vicious anger as the irrational fury of a frustrated toddler, of myself at the age of three or four, angry at having to wear dainty clothes and little white gloves and never being allowed to get dirty, throw a tantrum or simply be myself. That denied infantile rage, topped up with several decades' worth of repressed adult anger was bursting through now, flooding me with bad temper, aggression and sheer bloody malevolence, and I knew that I had to experience and release it all before recovering my balance.

Each fit of rage knocked off another piece of my self-image until I found to my relief that I had none left. That was marvellous. My old, hopelessly one-sided self-image had been due for recycling anyway and I was in no hurry to replace it until I got a better idea of the dark menagerie within that was still waiting to burst free. But between my rages I was beginning to enjoy great peace and joy and a fresh awareness of the basic rightness of things, including my own small existence. These spells of bliss corresponded to the physical well-being experienced between flare-ups, as if the drastic detoxification of the body was linked inseparably to a

parallel inner process which cast out, equally drastically, all my old, inappropriate negative emotions and
other poisonous residues. Both processes were as painful as they were necessary; both brought high rewards.

While experiencing this double shriving I also fished
around for additional therapies that might speed up my
recovery. After one or two failures, at a doctor friend's
recommendation I embarked on a series of weekly
treatments with Joe Corvo, the well-known zone therapist and healer. Despite his surname Joe turned out to
be a thoroughbred Yorkshireman, blessed with remarkable gifts; an ex-miner and trained opera singer turned
unorthodox therapist, attracting a large international
clientele. At our first meeting he explained his philosophy which sounded very similar to the Gerson principles. Disease, he said, was caused by the accumulation
of toxins in the body; health could only be restored by
removing all congestion, poisons and blockages. But,
unlike Gerson practitioners, Joe believed that the crys-
tallised toxins were deposited around the bunched
nerve endings in the feet (and to a lesser extent in the
hands, arms, head and back) and had to be broken up
by expert massage, which was his speciality. 'Once the
body's been cleared of toxins,' he told me, 'the disease
vanishes. But the true healing comes from the management above,' which was his code word for God. I had
no quarrel with either principle and asked him to go
ahead.

For several weeks Joe's treatment was excruciatingly
painful. Even the most gentle manipulation of the
pressure points on my sole, corresponding to liver,
kidneys, pancreas and lymphatic system, made me hiss,
squirm and beg for mercy – but only when he worked
on my right foot. The left one responded with no more
than mild discomfort. The contrast between the two
sides was striking; it confirmed Joe's opinion that my
fairly healthy left side was keeping the rest afloat.

In view of my agonised reaction to his massage, Joe

had to work slowly and patiently. But he brought miraculously fast results on the two occasions when I had accidentally damaged the eggshell-thin middle of my skin graft, causing wounds which I knew from the past would take up to six weeks to heal. On both occasions Joe gave me some carefully angled special massage, and to my amazement both wounds healed perfectly within forty-eight hours, instead of gaping and seeping for weeks, as they had done in the past. I was astounded and overjoyed. Joe did not understand what all the fuss was about. To be truly scientific, I should have deliberately damaged the skin graft for a third time and then kept away from Joe to see how long the wound took to heal, but we both felt that I had enough problems as it was.

Eventually the pain caused by Joe's steely yet gentle fingers diminished so much that I was able to keep up a normal conversation during treatment, with only an occasional yelp; clearly, the toxins were being broken up and eliminated. Sometimes, when I felt low, Joe sang for me throughout the session; sometimes he worked in total silence, engrossed in some intuitive reverie. Each treatment left me feeling better, clearer, more energetic. Throughout that long haul he was a great ally, helping my body to heal and boosting my often sagging confidence. I still go back to him for the odd maintenance treatment and tease him when even the strongest pressure from his wooden probe does not make me squirm.

The worst setback of that whole period occurred, ironically, on the second anniversary of my initial meeting with Mr Lennox, when I discovered a new swelling next to the tumour in my groin, a long, narrow, hard lump which threw me into total panic. Another tumour, I thought, breathless with shock: the melanoma has taken off and if it spreads now, in the tenth month of the therapy, nothing will stop it. I experienced the same overwhelming dread that I had felt when Mr Lennox had discovered the node in my groin. Once again I felt trapped and betrayed, this time by the therapy, betrayed and cruelly jolted out of my sense of safety and security. Oh no no, I keened inwardly, it can't be, can't be, I've kept the rules and never strayed, by now I should have at least half a renewed liver and sound organs to protect me . . . look here, Dr Gerson, this is not what you say in your book.

For a while even Hudie was caught up in my distress and desolation, but then we both calmed down and I got down to some fast telephoning. Charlotte, whom I managed to track down in California, ordered me back to the most intensive version of the therapy for at least three weeks. I groaned but obeyed, feeling like a model prisoner suddenly stripped of all her hard-earned privileges.

Dr Montague, who gave me an appointment at once, thought that the swelling might be nothing worse than a swollen lymph gland that was draining the tumour, but he admitted that he could not be sure without a biopsy which Charlotte had already vetoed. He quite agreed with that, because if the new swelling was cancerous, cutting it out would only spread the trouble. 'What counts ultimately,' Dr Montague said in his gentle, precise voice, 'is the patient's inner attitude and state of mind. Were you at peace with yourself before this swelling appeared?' I nodded. 'And your inner life . . . is your meditation going well?'

'Not as well as it should and certainly not regularly enough,' I admitted. 'Perhaps that's where I've gone wrong. Too much body and still not enough soul. Trying to get well as if my disease were purely physical when I know that it isn't. Oh, you know best how long I've been trying to put that right, but now it really can't wait any longer. If I don't break up this . . . dark night of the soul, my body will be in bad trouble again.' Bless you, I added inwardly, for being the kind of doctor to whom I can say this without fear of rejection or ridicule.

On the way home, poised between hope and despair, my mind remained blank. Only in the far background could I sense that familiar sigh. Oh my soul, remember past strivings, remember.

I needed help to reconnect with my inner resources. Catherine answered my distress call at once. She came along and guided me through the Simonton relaxation and visualising exercise which I had studiously neglected ever since first coming across it ten months before, concentrating instead on the physical therapy. Catherine recorded the exercise on a cassette so that I should be able to practise it without having to consult the instructions in the Simontons' book.

I kept up that exercise twice a day for two months, visualising my white blood cells in a variety of shapes – ferocious killer sharks, snarling dogs, tough little work-men with pneumatic drills – attacking and eliminating the tumour, which also appeared in different guises. The one that most amused me featured a packed mass of black slugs – highly appropriate, since slugs were the bane of my gardening life. The visualisation went very well. The tumour, however, refused to disappear or even shrink. This annoyed me, until I realised that the oncologist Dr Carl Simonton and his psychologist wife had developed their system for patients on orthodox cancer therapies, people who would equate the disap-pearance of the tumours with being cured. But we unorthodox Gersonites did not share that view; indeed, we knew that the body often encapsulated the tumour, building a sturdy container around it which was white-cell proof; for those reasons the visualisation was not likely to work for us in the projected way. However, by then I was convinced, at last, of the therapeutic value of visualisation, of using the imagination to reinforce bodily processes, and I did not want to lose it. So I modified the exercise, switching from tumour-bashing to a general boosting of the immune system and the vital organs. Did it help? I do not know. But the second

285

swelling, which had frightened me so dreadfully, was not followed by further lumps. After two months, when I felt that the visualisation work had served its purpose, I put it to rest.

But at the start of that process, around New Year's Day, Catherine also treated me to two sessions of guided imagery. They were regular marathons. Once we took the lid off my accumulated material, there was no end of stuff seeking expression in the form of vivid, powerful symbols, archetypal figures, bizarre and beautiful scenery and the thousand assorted images that the unconscious throws up with such precision, artistry and wit, if we tune in to it through the right techniques. 'You make a habit of saving my life once a year, around the New Year,' I said to Catherine after our second session. 'Last year you tracked down the Gerson therapy, now you're bailing out my psyche. What on earth can I say to you? "Thank you" sounds totally inadequate.' She shushed me and went on writing out her notes on the imagery which she wanted to leave with me for future reference. She looked every inch the professional therapist at work, yet the private person and unique friend within shone through, and I knew that she knew what I was trying to tell her.

The material that had emerged during those two sessions kept me at work for a long time. It was hard work, too, somewhat like sifting through the rubble of a landslide and trying to construct a garden out of it. As I went on, I was brought face to face with unknown and largely unacceptable facets of myself. I had to acknowledge faulty attitudes, sins of omission, a surprising degree of rigidity, fear of success, negative expectations and deep layers of denied sadness. The map of the psychological factors that had probably contributed to my illness began to take shape, only to lead me into ever deeper areas to explore. In the end I pieced together the graph of the life pattern that had inevitably led me towards disease, a graph that taught me enough for a couple of lifetimes. But that is another story.

The symbolic figures, brought into awareness through guided imagery, stayed with me until I assimilated their meaning. One of the toughest lessons of that process was to acknowledge my tendency to hang on to old hurts, long-dead conflicts, painful memories and other obsolete burdens, and to recognise how doggedly I was forcing myself to bear them, long after they had lost all relevance. Now I had to learn to let go of the past, just as I had recently learned to accept the present with all its limitations. Big deal, I thought tetchily; how elementary can my task get, how come that I have not mastered them long ago, despite my old familiarity with the theory of a sensible life? There was really no point in trying to answer that one.

In the course of relinquishing the shadows of the past I had to review and discard my old resentments, a necessity stressed by several unorthodox therapists who believe that nursing ancient resentments is a typical trait of the cancer-prone personality. The way they see it, resentment perpetuates the hurts of the past, complete with their full emotional charge, so that the old pain is relived again and again, accompanied by its original complement of stress, tension and depression, all of which act as a brake on the body's defences. Yes, that made sense; I embarked on the process at once. It took time and brought some vivid surprises, such as having to recognise that a number of my most resented hurts had been of my own making. But I persevered, and early one fine Sunday morning I completed the task to my satisfaction. Now there was no more bitterness left, not even towards two close friends who had rejected me so painfully all those years ago; I had set them, and myself, free, and felt all the better for it.

That morning Hudie took me for a drive to take advantage of the fleeting sunshine. As he slowed down to turn into a main road and then drove past a big hospital in central London, I happened to glance at the solitary figure standing outside the main entrance.

It was Mr Lennox.

Even in those few seconds I could see that he looked grey, tired and glum, with the beaten air of a man who lets his mask slip when he thinks he is unobserved. I gasped and buried my face in my hands. 'Yes, it's him,' Hudie said quietly. I was too shocked to speak. What stunned me was that in my determined drive to forgive, accept and release, I had forgotten – forgotten? – the one person towards whom I held the most enormous, most bitter resentment, whom I blamed every day of my life for having mutilated my body while leaving my disease unhealed, and, above all, for having shown me no scrap of sympathy or caring when I most needed it. How could I have overlooked him of all people? How honest and reliable was the rest of the work I had done?

What shocked me even more was the weird, uncanny coincidence, if that is what it was, that had made me glimpse Mr Lennox on the very morning when I thought I had dealt with my resentments once and for all. It had to be quite a hefty coincidence, too, for Hudie's car, out on a random drive, to pass that particular hospital on a Sunday morning just at the right moment for Mr Lennox to have left the building but not yet disappeared inside his car. The speed and precision with which my omission had been shown up reminded me of my childhood fantasies of instant divine retribution for misdeeds, with God's awesome majestic hand crashing through the classroom ceiling to slap His erring children. It was all too much, too dramatic, and I felt shattered. 'Don't cry, darling,' Hudie said gently, mis-interpreting my tears, 'you don't have to go back to him ever again.' I could not explain why I was weeping and simply accepted his comforting touch on my arm. But in the weeks to come it took me much time and considerable pain to resolve my one-sided inner conflict with Mr Lennox and to accept, without rancour, that he had only done his job by his own lights and that it was futile to blame him for being what he was, a product of his training and professional limitations. When at last I was able to feel pity for his sad, beaten look on that Sunday morning – had he just lost a patient or suffered a personal blow? – I knew that at last I had completed the job.

Much else happened on the inner plane during those final months. The breakthrough came with the realisation that neither the cancer nor my recovery were the most important things in my life, that both were parts of my pattern but not the pattern itself, and that it was time for me to look through wider windows. Outwardly all went on as before. My body produced no more lumps and continued to grow fitter and stronger. I still disliked the restrictions of the gradually reducing therapy, I still swore and growled when my helper let me down, or the carrots arrived a day late, or the need to make another juice filled me with terminal boredom. But the perspective and the resonance had changed and I was slowly moving from the dark depths, towards the surface again.

My contacts with the American patients I had met in Mexico were flimsy and I suspected that soon they would cease altogether: they all hated writing letters, and to keep in touch by telephone, which was their preferred method, was too expensive. But I did get a long letter from my friend Carl, announcing that he had his tumour removed at a famous Californian hospital He enclosed a copy of the biopsy report which made fascinating reading once I had cracked the code of the medical jargon. According to the report, Carl's lump contained some dead melanoma cells; the remaining live ones, looking atypical – battered by the therapy? – were sandwiched between layers of connective tissue, and the whole growth was neatly contained in a two-millimetre thick capsule, purpose-built by the body to hold the malignancy in custody. 'I was convinced before

I had it removed that it was going to take years to dissolve,' Carl wrote. 'The encasement would probably have continued to grow thicker, which is the way my body apparently chose to fight the cancer. The surgeon did a real plastic surgery job on the scar and I was very pleased all round,' he added in his usual laconic way.

Some months later, having returned home from Clinic Del Sol, Carl sent me a long recorded message, with full details of his diet and lifestyle, adapted to the toxic non-Gerson world. He had completely recovered as he had always said he would, and I celebrated his victory quietly but delightedly. Another cause for celebration came in October 1981, when fifty healed patients, previously written off as incurables, attended a convention honouring the centenary of Dr Gerson's birth. Just knowing that they were all there under one roof in San Diego, hale and well and wearing their battle scars instead of medals, boosted my morale enormously.

I also received news of losses. Doris, the black ex-nurse was dead. Flora, the old lady who had been recovering so well from her senile afflictions, slipped right back into them when she went home from the clinic, because her family found it impossible to keep her on the demanding therapy. One month on ordinary supermarket food and no Gerson routine made her relapse into mumbling, mindless senility. There was also the case of the young woman whom I met at La Gloria when she was still full of cancer but beginning to improve. She died some time afterwards of unrelated causes, and at the autopsy was found to be clear of cancer; a truly pyrrhic victory.

I kept regularly in touch with Charlotte, sending her my blood test results and asking countless questions. As the end of the intensive therapy drew near, Charlotte sent me some dietary guidelines. 'When your eighteen months are up,' she wrote, 'don't jump into steak and kidney pie. Be sensible, cut down on the juices gradually, add proteins carefully, watch your uric acid. And never, never go back to eating salt. You don't want to go through all this again.' She was right: I did not.

To mark the end of my year and a half on the strict therapy I gave a small party for my closest friends and allies who had kept me going throughout that embattled period. It was a warm, funny, colourful evening that made my house come to life again after its long seclusion. At one stage Catherine and I withdrew to my bedroom for a few quiet moments of private celebration. We sat down, looked at each other, opened our mouths and then shut them again simultaneously; just for once neither of us knew what to say.

'Well, well,' said Catherine when we had recovered from that unaccustomed moment of speechlessness. 'When you came back from Mexico, I promised to monitor your progress and let you know from time to time how I thought you were doing. Congratulations, my love – I think you've made it and that you're doing extremely well. I hope you're as delighted with your progress as I am.'

'Oh yes,' I said, 'absolutely delighted. But I've this silly feeling of having followed a kind of inside-out and upside-down scenario. What I mean is that a good story should have a nice slow start, building up to a busy middle full of action and excitement, and then lead on to a grand finale, happy or otherwise. But with me all the drama and the action got crammed into the early phases, and all that came afterwards was the tedious, plodding part of the journey. Even that's going to fizzle out now, with no sign of a suitable ending.'

'I see,' said Catherine thoughtfully. 'I suppose as a writer you would have preferred a better story line.'

'Well, yes. And especially a different ending. I'm delighted to feel so fit and well, but I would have liked a little extra, something definite and dramatic . . . like regaining a lost sense or throwing away crutches or surgical supports or whatever, just to make a proper ending to the story.'

Catherine pondered this for a moment. 'I suppose you could always burn your enema bucket in Piccadilly Circus,' she suggested. 'But anyway, what makes you think that your story needs a proper ending? As far as I'm concerned, it's just about to begin.'

17

CATHERINE WAS RIGHT. Ends and beginnings are inseparable, time is seamless; the only thing to do about milestones is to salute them and walk on. Our brief exchange that evening was a milestone in itself, as well as a celebration of our tried and tested friendship. From then onwards I moved steadily though warily towards a more normal lifestyle, going out regularly without feeling the hourly tug of the invisible cord that had tied me to the juicer for so long. It was time for thanksgiving and for starting to rebuild my life, for I felt sure that my long journey through sickness, struggle and recovery was over at last.

By the time I was virtually off the therapy, except for sticking to a sensible diet and drinking one large juice a day, I no longer gave a thought to my tumour that was sitting quietly and unchangingly in my groin. It was so hard to the touch that Mr Montague and I habitually referred to it as Little Rock. He thought it had probably become encapsulated, perhaps even calcified, and I gladly went along with that view. One day Margaret Straus told me that my case history did not qualify for inclusion among those of recently recovered 'incurable' Gerson patients, because, having refused a second biopsy, I had no proof of having had secondary melanoma. This made me feel somewhat peeved. Granted, I said to her, I had no medically acceptable proof, yet I did not think that my case could be dismissed as merely anecdotal, since I still had the secondary tumour itself and that should be evidence enough. Ah yes, said

Margaret, but they could only present fully documented cases, and on the whole a typed pathology report was easier to handle than a built-in tumour. Yes, she had a point there. Sometimes I wondered myself whether keeping the tumour in my groin was not an unduly eccentric way to store my medical record, and I vaguely decided to have it removed one day. But for the time being there was no hurry.

And then, in November 1983, my tumour began to grow. I first noticed its increased size one evening in the bath, which is the usual place for discovering ominous bodily changes. My reaction was puzzlement, not fear. As far as I could tell, Little Rock had no conceivable medical, dietary or psychological cause to get out of control. Besides, was it really growing or was I imagining things?

It was, and I was not. By mid-January there could be no doubt about its slow but steady increase. Now I was really baffled. I was feeling as fit and strong as ever, looking healthy and bouncing with energy; surely that was not the condition of someone with a newly activated cancer? But apprehension began to seep in. One evening I recalled ruefully how I had complained to Catherine eighteen months before about the undramatic ending of my Gerson saga. Was the tumour going to provide a dramatic and possibly devastating finale at this late stage?

Oh no, it was not. I would not let it. By way of fighting back I launched into concentrated visualisation twice a day, willing the tumour to shrink. After three days the groin area and part of my thigh turned inflamed and stayed so for a whole week. That was highly interesting, because in Gerson terms an inflammation is a favourable sign which often precedes the softening and shrinking of tumours. Moreover, it seemed to prove that by strong mental programming I was able to trigger the correct healing mechanism in my body. And that was splendid. The only trouble was that Little Rock, bulging boldly, remained unchanged.

As I could not do the job myself, I went to see Dr Montague. He looked me over and found me in good working order, but had to admit that Little Rock had grown bigger. As puzzled as myself, he suggested a scan of the pelvic area. Even though some radiation was involved, he felt that was the only way to find out what was happening. I bristled a little. Melanoma, I knew, was radiation-sensitive, but I agreed to the scan, since there was no alternative.

I also wrote to Charlotte to report the situation. My lifestyle had not changed, I explained, except that since the previous autumn I had been taking calcium and magnesium tablets at a knowledgeable friend's suggestion, to protect myself from brittle bones later in life. Apart from that small extra I had been following her instructions faithfully. Could she suggest any reason for the lump growing bigger?

Charlotte replied promptly, but her letter brought me no cheer. For one thing she reminded me of a passage in her father's book which clearly stated that calcium and other minerals were not to be taken by cancer patients, because in some cases they could cause tumours to regrow. For another she advised me to go back on the full intensive therapy, complete with thirteen juices, five enemas, medication, the lot. 'This should last at least three months,' she wrote, 'or until your tumour is reduced and softened – or gone. This is what would happen to you if you were to come back to La Gloria, with the addition of ozone treatment.' She ended her letter with a cheery greeting – 'You'll get ahead of it again, don't worry.'

At that moment even a thunderbolt from Zeus would not have shaken me more than Charlotte's reply. I looked up The Book, felt like kicking myself for having forgotten Dr Gerson's taboo on mineral supplements, flung all my tablets in the dustbin and sat down to do some hard thinking. The one thing I knew with certainty was that I could not run the full therapy at home for a single week, let alone three months or more, for I would not be able to cope with its demands either physically or psychologically, and that some other solution would have to be found.

Hudie was the only person who knew about this latest twist, which he regarded with equanimity, convinced that there was nothing seriously wrong with me. I then informed my mother, Catherine, John and two more close friends, asking them to keep the news to themselves. At this stage I wanted to keep it from everyone else, especially from my contacts in the alternative therapy field, because I suspected that they would fear the worst and write me off as another cancer victim who had lost her battle. And I had no intention of letting that happen.

It was quite a relief when the time came for my pelvic scan. It took forty minutes and passed uneventfully. When it was over, the woman consultant radiologist who had supervised the scan from the technician's booth, came in to see me. 'The pictures are still coming through from the computer,' she said, 'but I've seen the first few. Your tumour is completely encapsulated – it's most interesting. And there's no sign of any abnormality anywhere.'

'You mean the cancer hasn't spread?'

'That's right. The tumour is well defined and it's all on its own.'

'Oh, good,' I said, sending an inward salute to Dr Gerson's memory. 'Can you see what's inside the lump?'

She smiled. 'No, I'm afraid that's impossible. But would you mind telling me about this therapy you've been following? I gather from your doctor that it's rather . . . unusual.'

Still lying on the hard, unyiedling plastic table of the scanning room, I gave her a brief summary of the

296

therapy. But all along part of my mind was dancing around the good news: Little Rock was encapsulated, solitary and well defined, and that made its inexplicable growth less worrying.

The results of the scan, two large sheets of X-ray pictures and the consultant's report, which Dr Montague handed over to me, reassured me even more. The consultant expressed the view that the tumour was resectable, in other words amenable to surgical removal. The pictures, twenty in all, showed astounding land-scapes and abstract compositions in black and grey which, I realised, represented the contents of my abdo-men and pelvic area. They were fascinating images, yet I could not warm to them or feel even a spark of ownership, even though I knew that the neat twin objects appearing in several pictures were my kidneys, and that the bold and pleasing arc surrounding a thicket of shadowy parts was, in fact, my pelvis. It was all most interesting, but all I had eyes for was the tumour, Little Rock unveiled at last, nestling in my right groin like Humpty Dumpty before his great fall. It was rounded, around five centimetres across, and it sat uncompromis-ingly on its own. Somewhere between the size of a golf and a tennis ball, it had certainly grown plump and stately since Mr Lennox first discovered it three years before.

'So far so good,' I said to Dr Montague, 'now at least I know where I am. But where do I go from here? Should I have this thing removed?'

He gazed at his note pad and said, 'I don't think I can answer that question. On the whole I am not in favour of surgery in such cases, but with an encapsulated tumour like yours perhaps it would be safe. I'd like to know what the Gerson people think.'

'So would I. I'll find out and let you know,' I promised.

But for a few days I did nothing about it and went on with my ordinary daily life, as if waiting for some sign or omen to prod me into action. No sign appeared. At least on the conscious level all was quiet. But one evening I suddenly experienced an influx of energy, for want of a better term, that was like a mild electric shock, startling but painless, and I knew that there was nothing else to wait for, the moment to act had come. What is more, I also knew what I had to do.

I rang Charlotte in California, reported on the result of the scan, and asked her whether she thought I should have the encapsulated tumour removed. 'Yes, I think that's a good idea,' she replied, 'provided that afterwards you go on the strict therapy for a few weeks. And of course you must choose your surgeon carefully. But the main thing is the intensive therapy after the operation. If you can set that up once more at home . . .'

'No, I can't.' One deep breath and then the plunge. 'I should like to return to La Gloria, have the lump removed by one of your approved surgeons and then stay on the intensive therapy for a couple of weeks. That way I can't go wrong, can I?'

'Certainly not.' Charlotte sounded pleased. 'That would be the best possible way to do it and finish off the whole business properly. When do you want to come? And how long can you stay?'

'Two weeks at the utmost. What with the air fare I can't even afford that, but I'll manage somehow.' There goes my nest egg, I thought. Little Rock was becoming as expensive as a good diamond. We fixed the date of my arrival and said *au revoir*. Reluctant though I was to return to Mexico, I relished the prospect of seeing Charlotte again. Dr Montague, whom I informed at once, expressed his approval. Provided I was to be under the care of Gerson physicians and operated on by a surgeon of their choice, he had no objection.

Making arrangements for my trip smacked of here-we-go-again familiarity. Once again it was Gatwick to San Diego, except that now, in March 1984, I was fit, robust and pink-cheeked, a world away from my gravely ill, grey-faced self in January 1981. Also, I travelled light, with my second smallest suitcase. This time, I had told Hudie, I would be back very soon.

I arrived at La Gloria at dinner time. The unmistakable, powerful aroma of the Hippocrates soup hit me as I walked into the well-known dining-room. The world may turn somersaults, I thought with amusement, galaxies may rise and fall, but wherever Gerson patients foregather, the Hippocrates soup bubbles on. I joined a group at a large table. My pale, nervous neighbour asked me whose visitor I was, since she could see that I was not a patient. 'As a matter of fact I'm a former patient,' I admitted, 'back for a refresher.' And I left it at that.

On the following morning the clinic's precise non-stop routine engulfed me once more and I went along with it, even though I felt a bit of a cheat among so many sick people. Charlotte arrived, looking as fresh and vigorous as ever. I had a long talk with her, and later with Dr Arturo who was to look after me. In the afternoon he brought along Dr Ricardo, the surgeon whom he had chosen to operate on me. Dr Ricardo, who was keenly interested in the Gerson therapy, examined my tumour and then studied the scan pictures at length. The operation, he said, would have to take place at his Tijuana hospital, not in La Gloria's smallish operating room, and he would use the nerve block technique instead of a general anaesthetic which, according to the Gerson credo, played hell with the immune system.

'Congratulations,' Dr Ricardo said at the conclusion of our conversation. 'You've beaten the statistics.'

'What do you mean?'

'Well, patients with secondary malignant melanoma normally last only six to eight months,' he said cheerfully. 'You're doing pretty well.'

We next met in the operating theatre of a splendid

new hospital in unlovely Tijuana. The surgery took ninety minutes and made me feel very lonely, because although I was fully conscious, I could not understand a word of the merry Spanish conversation that ebbed and flowed between Dr Ricardo, his fellow surgeon, the anaesthetist and several nurses. They talked fast, in lively, amused tones and they laughed a lot, all of which made me feel dreadfully excluded. Come on, I thought, I should like to share your jokes, too, and besides, why is the job taking so long? 'How are we doing?' I occasionally asked Dr Ricardo, longing to be let in on the act, but all I got were general reassurances and no details. Once or twice the anaesthetist, who had beautiful brown eyes, held my hand to comfort me, and that was nice. I felt no pain, only pressure in the groin area.

Suddenly a nurse appeared by my side and showed me something in a metal dish. It was the tumour, an oval, whitish-yellow object the size of a child's fist, as smooth and whole as a new rubber ball. 'So that's what it's like,' I said stupidly to the nurse who spoke no English – but then is there any appropriate way in any language to greet one's newly removed tumour? Little Rock swam into my field of vision once more, this time imprisoned in a glass jar, presumably on its way to the pathologist. It felt odd to see it disappear for ever.

'A most interesting case,' Dr Ricardo said when it was all over and I had been transferred to a trolley. 'This tumour of yours wasn't attached to its surroundings like normal tumours which grow into muscles and organs and link up with blood vessels; it just lay there, as if it had been waiting to be lifted out. There was only one point of attachment,' he went on in his slightly halting American English, 'to a blood vessel, which I had to deal with. And of course I had to reconnect the lymph nodes, too, and all that took some time. But such a free-standing tumour is unusual. And the capsule is unusually thick and tough. We'll know more about that when we get the pathologist's report. How are you feeling?'

'Fine. No complaints,' I said truthfully. If he had not instructed me not to walk for a couple of days, I would have risen from the trolley, got dressed and asked to be driven back to La Gloria. As it was, I had to spend the night in the hospital – and nearly starve, because the only food on offer was a cup of purple jelly and a glass of milk, both of which I had to refuse. But even that did not matter, nor did the slight post-operative pain. The major part of my mission had been completed. The rest, I felt sure, would be easy.

Back at La Gloria, Dr Arturo added the ozone treatment to my crowded schedule. Ozone, he explained, had been routinely used in several European countries and in South America for a long time. The Gerson clinic had introduced it in 1983, since which time the chances of even very advanced cases had improved. 'Ozone kills bacteria, viruses and fungi on contact,' he said. 'It increases oxygenation in the body, which, as you know, is very important with cancer patients, and through that extra oxygenation it's able to destroy tumour tissue.'

That was wonderful, I said warily, but did he think that I had any tumour tissue left that needed to be destroyed? 'Not at all,' he replied. 'I want you to have ozone as a matter of routine after your operation, just to make sure that everything's clear and to give you a boost. That extra oxygen is good even for perfectly fit people – just ask Charlotte, she's tried it herself.' The twice-daily intravenous ozone injections undoubtedly boosted my well-being. They also threw me into a coma of boredom, since they had to be administered excru-tiatingly slowly, to avoid pushing a bubble into the bloodstream. And since the nurses spoke very little English, ozone-time was long, immobile and sadly mute. But it did not matter. All was well, the incision was healing very fast and soon I would be going home.

The pathologist's report arrived when I was already up and about, feeling extremely well. It described the tumour's appearance in detail and went on to say that this well-defined encapsulated growth contained extensive necrosed – dead – tissue, and also clusters of metastasized melanoma cells.

The last line stunned me. As I stared at it, a great, dark chill closed in on me and shut out the world. Clusters of cancer cells, I thought in a panic, *live* melanoma cells after all those years on the therapy? Good God, in that case I had never really recovered, never beaten my illness – or had I? I could no longer think properly. All I knew was that this was my worst disappointment ever, a bitter defeat. I could not handle it and did not wish to fight any more. In those few minutes of shock my future seemed to evaporate. All I had left was the certainty of defeat.

Charlotte entered at that very moment and received the full force of my despair. I thrust the report at her, biting back my tears, but she told me that she had already seen it. 'Well then, it's no good, is it?' I blurted out. 'This is it. I'm a failure of the therapy, you can write me off. If after all these years I still have live melanoma cells . . .'

'Hold it,' she cut in. 'What on earth are you talking about?' I blew my nose mournfully and shrugged. '*You* had no live melanoma cells, your encapsulated tumour contained some; that's a different matter altogether. You're a success of the therapy, not a failure.'

'It doesn't look like that to me,' I said sulkily.

'Oh, come on. Surely you know how fast melanoma spreads once it has metastasized, don't you?' I nodded. 'Well, your secondary was found over three years ago, you went on the therapy and produced no further lumps, you came off the therapy some time ago and produced no further lumps, you're alive and well, and your tumour had a fifteen-millimetre thick capsule around it.'

302

'Fifteen? That's almost bulletproof!'

'Exactly. And now it's all gone and you're in great shape. So how can you say you're a failure?'

'Ah, but those live cells? Why did they stay alive?'

Charlotte sighed. 'Probably because the capsule protected them,' she said patiently, 'so that the tumour-killing elements of the therapy couldn't get through to the centre.' She sketched a model of Little Rock in the air, to emphasise her point. 'Don't forget, the capsule consists of benign tissue which is fairly normal in composition, and so the immune system doesn't recognise it as alien matter that has to be destroyed. It's no accident that the live cells were deep inside the capsule, surrounded by all the dead tissue.'

My brain began to function again. 'What you mean is that the capsule worked both ways,' I said tentatively. 'It kept the cancer in and the therapy out, at least to some extent. In other words you can't win.'

'But you have won,' Charlotte replied. 'Your body did the right thing all along. It defended itself most effectively. Please stop this nonsense about being a failure. Why don't you celebrate your success instead?' She smiled and left to continue with her rounds.

I was still trying to sort out my confusion when Dr Arturo walked in, looking pleased. Both the surgeon and the pathologist had found my case highly unusual, he said. He himself had seen similar encapsulated tumours in Gerson patients, predominantly dead lumps that could be lifted out easily, with only minimal cutting. 'One of them belonged to a melanoma patient,' he said, 'whom you may remember. He was here during your first stay.'

'Oh, you mean my old friend Carl,' I exclaimed. 'Yes. I know about his operation, he sent me a copy of his biopsy report at the time.'

'Well, he's been very well ever since,' Dr Arturo went on. 'And we've had other similar cases, too. If the body isn't able to destroy and eliminate the cancer cells through the usual channels, then it surrounds and isolates them. The same process is at work when people have a bullet, a nail or a piece of shrapnel in their bodies for twenty years without even knowing about it, until one day it begins to hurt and then it's discovered and removed. The only difference is that with cancer the body needs the therapy in order to do the job.'

I pondered that for a moment. 'Yes, that makes sense. But why was my lump growing bigger?'

'I don't know. Perhaps as the malignant cells died off in the middle they grew hard and became part of the outer capsule. That might have made the tumour bulkier. Or perhaps all that calcium you've been taking was used by your body to make the capsule even thicker. We'll never know for sure.'

'And what would have happened if I hadn't had it removed?'

'I guess eventually all the cells would have died and you would have been left with a hard, lifeless lump. Since your immune system has been working very well, that's a strong possibility. But all that is theory. The lump's gone, you've nothing else to worry about.'

He was right. Gradually I recovered my calm, but it took me some time to understand the full significance of my experience and to realise that it was a victory, not a defeat. Those live cells inside the tumour reinforced the validity of my story instead of spoiling it. Moreover, they were the ultimate proof and vindication of the therapy.

The Gerson method, I now saw, had not only brought under control my highly malignant, fast-moving cancer and stopped it from doing further damage, which is a great deal more than what orthodox treatment could have achieved; it had also raised my immune system to such a high level of efficiency that I had been able to lead an active, increasingly full life with those potentially lethal live cells surviving inside the tumour, held fast and rendered powerless by my body's defences. It was rather like having violent murderers living in my house, safely imprisoned in a stout escape-proof chamber that made them both harmless and unnoticeable.

Both the process and its outcome were so different from the methods and results of orthodox cancer medicine that I found it hard to think of them along parallel lines. 'The trouble is,' I said to Charlotte shortly before my return to London, 'that here at La Gloria my experience sounds fairly routine, but anywhere else it would sound crazy or even unbelievable. If I told an orthodox cancer specialist that I'd been marching around for three years and two months with live melanoma cells in my groin and that they'd been no trouble at all, he would probably refer me to the nearest psychiatrist.'

'Ah,' Charlotte said with a mischievous smile, 'but you'd have the pathologist's report and a slide of your tumour to prove your story.'

'That's true.' And then a thought struck me. 'Listen,' I said urgently, 'now that I have all this medically acceptable evidence, will you include me among the case histories of recovered Gerson patients?'

'Yes, I think I will,' said Charlotte.

18

CHARLOTTE WAS AS good as her word. My name has been added to the Gerson list of 'cured incurables'; I have even been included among the twenty 'best cases' submitted to the scrutiny of independent American medical authorities. Whatever happens to me in the future – and I take great care not to fall under buses – nothing can strike me off the Gerson register.

Since coming off the therapy, which now seems a lifetime ago, I have done a lot of hard thinking, trying to draw general conclusions from my particular experience, and in the process my ideas have undergone a drastic change.

At one stage, in the first flush of recovered health and well-being, my most urgent concern was to see the Gerson therapy officially accepted, widely practised and as freely available as orthodox treatments are in Britain today. It has always distressed me that patients without adequate funds have no access to the Gerson programme. I thought that the only task ahead was to break through medical prejudice and create the right conditions for proving the potential of the therapy, subjecting it to proper scientific scrutiny and objective assessment. If the dietary treatment of cancer and other chronic diseases were carried out in large-scale, impeccably conducted pilot schemes, I felt sure that recovery rates would soar, a new era would start in medicine, all would be well.

Today I see things somewhat differently.

My basic tenets are unchanged. I know that dietary

therapy works. I believe that there will be no real breakthrough in the treatment of the killer diseases of civilisation until food is recognised as the most basic vital key to health, the main womb-to-tomb factor that determines our well-being, energy level, resistance to disease, state of mind, behaviour, rate of ageing and lifespan. In the light of what is already known about the impact of nutrition, it seems crazy to try and tackle chronic degenerative diseases without analysing minutely patients' eating habits – and knowing how to correct them. Yet that is happening today. The doctors' only excuse is ignorance. Nutrition is barely touched upon in medical training.

I suspect that medicine's corporate indifference to diet springs from the probably unformulated *macho* view that diet equals food equals kitchen equals woman's work, and that makes it inferior by definition and unworthy of scientific interest. In other words, food is yet another feminine value that has been degraded and banished from its proper place by our overweeningly masculine order. Now it must be restored. Doctors will have to learn how to use diet as a tool of prevention and healing, if only to keep up with their better-educated patients and with the growing number of non-medical practitioners who already use dietary therapy successfully.

In that early phase, I believed that once doctors had broken through their indifference barrier, they would realise that nutrition is too important to be left to the profit-centred processing industry whose heavily advertised junk foods actually create an overfed but undernourished population. I felt sure that doctors would take the lead in questioning the use of the countless chemical additives whose cumulative effects are unknown, and in denouncing the appalling meals served in so many hospitals, schools and old people's homes. Some doctors, I thought, might even consider the possibility of treating addiction and rehabilitating the old through correct feeding, since conventional approaches achieve very little in those two topical areas. Enlightened doctors would have a great deal to do, I felt. They might even stop living on junk foods themselves and improve their health.

Today I can see that this was a dizzily ambitious scenario. Little wonder it did not work out. The increasing public concern over additives and food adulteration was sparked off not by the medical profession (yet 'doctor' means teacher), but by environmental groups and small, impecunious organisations like the Soil Association. Bestselling books on additives by non-medical authors alerted the lay public to the tricks and half-truths of food labelling, sparking off the scrutiny of the small print on tins and boxes which quickly became a favourite supermarket sport among intelligent lay shoppers. A small group of radical writers on food and nutrition, headed by Geoffrey Cannon, Derek Cooper, James Erlichman, Barbara Griggs, Leslie Kenton and, last but not least, the late Caroline Walker, have exposed the half-truths, euphemisms and cynical antics of the food processing industry to a wide audience. Only a very small number of medical doctors and nutritionists have tried to influence the Government's food policy, largely in vain. The medical profession as a whole has remained indifferent.

Yet even if all this changed tomorrow and doctors became the front-line champions of healthy nutrition, our problems would only be eased, not solved, for we would still be up against a poisoned ecosystem which is in turn poisoning us.

The extent of the disaster is only beginning to emerge, as the many, apparently separate, global disease symptoms meet and merge into a single eco-catastrophe. It is as if a lot of small and unconnected grass fires suddenly flared up and united in one huge conflagration, threatening to engulf us all.

In the early Seventies when, as a far-out fringe

element, I first realised how grossly we were mismanaging the Earth, I used to fear a great backlash from Nature – tidal waves, floods, earthquakes, tornadoes, climatic disasters – as a reaction to our greed and stupidity. Some of it is happening already, with the dangers of the damaged ozone layer and the Greenhouse Effect brooding on the near horizon.

Yet all that is only the outer half of the story.

The inner half is worse: it is the natural backlash that is already taking place in our bodies which sicken as a result of our global self-poisoning. Nature need not unleash any old-fashioned plague to teach us a lesson. We have already created our own epidemics of cancer, heart disease and a whole batch of other chronic degenerative diseases. And, of course, AIDS.

The meaning of that abbreviation – Acquired Immune Deficiency Syndrome – holds the key to other chronic diseases, too. The root cause of all our health problems is self-inflicted immune deficiency which makes the body helpless against disease-causing factors.

Scientists searching for the cause of the epidemic that is killing North Sea seals, besides threatening dolphins, whales and other forms of marine life, have pinpointed a virus which, they believe, has been present in the environment for a long time, without causing harm. But now that the seals' immune defences have been gravely weakened by the worsening pollution of the North Sea, they succumb to the virus in their hundreds.

The explanation is as plausible as it is tragic.

But why stop at marine creatures?

Read 'humans' for seals and 'Western countries' for North Sea, and you have the explanation for the rampaging cancer epidemic, affecting ever-younger age-groups and estimated to hit one in three in the overall population. The human immune system, just as that of the seals, has developed over millions of years to cope with any danger arising from its natural environment. It was not designed to deal with the myriad man-made factors that attack it in our de-natured modern habitat, factors ranging from pollution, radiation and electro-magnetic disturbances to ubiquitous toxic chemicals, noise, stress, bad nutrition, the ravages of alcohol, tobacco and street drugs, and of the over-lavishly pre-scribed antibiotics and other medical drugs which leave toxic residues in the body.

Weakened by this unprecedented and permanent onslaught of harmful substances, the immune system can hardly be expected to do its original job properly and cope, for instance, with the large number of malig-nant cells which our bodies produce every day as a matter of routine, not to mention the many other enemies of health and survival.

Why stop at the seals, indeed?

In a chilling way, our global self-poisoning is just like cancer: it has reached an advanced stage without obvious and unambiguous symptoms, and now that it is at last being diagnosed, it may be too late for treatment. Just like the human body, the Earth is a complex organism of finely tuned and interdependent systems, and today, just like any cancer patient, it is suffering from severe pollution and destructive, soil-starving farming methods. While that situation contin-ues, even a fundamental reform of medicine would not make much difference.

Sick soil, sick food plants and animals, sick people: the cycle is inescapable. Max Gerson's restrained obser-vations of sixty years ago are a shattering critique of our lifestyle of today. In 1930 he forecast a steep rise in cancer and other degenerative diseases unless agricul-ture reverted to natural methods. 'Organic food seems to be the answer to the cancer problem,' he wrote six decades ago. It is not hard to guess what he would say today if he saw the lifeless, ravaged soils of the devel-oped countries where so much of the world's grain is grown, and the swelling load of toxic chemicals which food plants are made to bear and pass on to us. And, once again, our doctors have failed us. Whenever organic and conventional farmers argue in public, they do so in terms of respective yields and costs. Human health, which should be the doctors' concern, is barely mentioned.

Yet there is ample fresh evidence to show that only organically farmed soil contains all the minerals, trace elements, enzymes, micro-organisms and other substances that are necessary to maintain health. To quote just one eloquent example, the amino-acid methionine, needed to clear heavy metal residues from the body, is present in organically farmed soil only, which is why nutritional therapists have to prescribe it in capsule form for patients in need of detoxification.

The self-poisoning process is becoming faster and more severe. We have known for a long time that the body fat of most animals, from Arctic penguins to humans in big cities, contains insecticide residues, and that some herbicides are more damaging to people than to weeds. Now we also know that carcinogenic nitrates, derived from nitrogenous fertilizers, are infesting our streams and rivers, killing off aquatic life, and seeping inexorably towards our ground water supplies; once they get there, no power can remove them. Earth, air, fresh and salt water are all polluted and poisoned.

What is the point of spending huge sums on more and better hospitals, expensive early diagnosis equipment, complex research projects and ever stronger, ever costlier drugs if at the same time we add carcinogens to our drinking water, toxic chemicals to our soil and air, and a rich variety of rubbish to our already deficient food? Have the decision-makers completely forgotten the simple link between cause and effect?

Once you have thought through this schizoid situation, it is no longer possible to remain silent about it.

Yet that is only the agricultural-nutritional side of the self-poisoning picture. The industrial and nuclear sides are even more sinister. The authorities keep assuring the public that despite Chernobyl and the regularly surfacing faults, accidents, near-misses and clusters of cancers plaguing nuclear power stations, all is well and safe; but despite expensive advertising campaigns and PR exercises a growing sector of the public does not believe a word of it. The protestations of experts are all too predictable and lacking in credibility, since no one on Earth can prove the long-term safety and harmlessness of nuclear power. Besides, even the problem of radioactive waste disposal has not been solved.

The same technique of empty reassurance, followed by a hasty upward adjustment of safety limits, applies to toxic industrial processes. In the end, though, the objectors normally win some concessions. But why should there be a kind of bizarre contest between polluters who are in the business of making money, and ordinary people anxious to salvage our common habitat? And how much more environmental damage is needed for the decision-makers to notice the link between our increasingly toxic world and our worsening collective health?

If the wholesomeness of a habitat is mirrored in the health of its population, then the developed world does not score very well. An increased lifespan is a dubious blessing if old people spend their extra time on Earth crippled by arthritis, stricken with cancer or reduced to mindless senility.

In a grim way it helps that the human animal itself is becoming an endangered species. The threatened extinction of other creatures has so far inspired the public to raise funds, but not to make a connection between vanishing wildlife and ailing humans. Now that our own health and survival are at risk, perhaps people will wake up and act.

They had better do so. At present we cannot expect much help from the official custodians of our well-being. Medicine's interest in our increasingly self-poisoned environment is moderate and largely theoretical. In the vivid phrase of that great medical maverick,

Denis Burkitt, 'These days doctors keep mopping up the floor instead of turning off the tap that causes the flooding, but then,' he adds, 'you get paid more for mopping up.'

Governments will not turn off the tap, either. They encourage the very practices – chemicalised agriculture and industrial-nuclear expansion – which cause much of the damage. Not upsetting important interest groups that create wealth and employment – food processing, the road lobby, the chemical and pharmaceutical giants, and so on – is seen as more important than facing the nation's basic health problems. Governments also ignore and even silence the occasional authoritative voice that criticises the status quo. Politicians are interested in the cost of health care, but do not understand its economics. And, in any case, Governments are too short-lived to feel committed to people's long-term well-being.

If we want change, we must bring it about ourselves. There is no reason why we should wait for some paternalistic official voice to dictate our lifestyle. Ever since my first return from Mexico in 1981, I have been thinking in terms of individual action, grass root effort, self-help and personal responsibility: the same kind of do-it-yourself commitment which makes the therapy go round, only on a much wider scale. Today there are more and more people who have found ways to lead a saner, less poisoned kind of life and who help others to do the same. I suspect that if Max Gerson were alive today, he would feel more at home among organic farmers, Greens, alternative therapists and lay seekers of health than among his medical colleagues.

We must introduce consumerism, by which I mean the freedom to make informed choices that serve our best interests, into the two areas that really matter: food production and medicine. Oddly enough, these are the two areas where we, as consumers, have very little choice; but until now we have not asked for it. Yet the food we eat and the medical care we get are the two pillars on which our quality of life rests. To change them for the better would be a fundamental revolution.

Can the change be brought about? I do not know. Sometimes the task seems as hopeless as trying to demolish a mountain with a nail file. But that is a passing impression. What I perceive more relevantly is that there is something different in the air; perhaps the foretaste of an idea whose time has come. I am not naïve enough to overestimate small signs or to believe that a hundred compost bins in suburban organic gardens can temper the environmental damage caused by a single trainload of agro-chemicals; nor do I imagine that powerless individuals of goodwill can succeed against the big battalions – at least not at once. But I do believe that the tide is turning and that the whole is more than the sum of its parts, and I intend to live long enough to see the new paradigm that will emerge from today's sick, sad mess. Meanwhile I shall follow the rules which I learnt in the carrot juice years – live from day to day, do what you can, remember what you want, and get on with it.

Postscript

THE DIETARY PRINCIPLES of Dr Gerson add up to an excellent programme for the prevention of disease which anyone can follow. The average Western diet is under increasingly sharp critical scrutiny at present, and the unbreakable link between nutrition and disease is fast gaining acceptance among thinking people. Quite a few of Dr Gerson's original discoveries of fifty or more years ago are being 're-discovered' now by doctors and researchers.

For instance, in June 1983 the American National Academy of Sciences published guidelines on how to reduce cancer risks by nutrition. Their main recommendations included a drastic reduction in the intake of all kinds of fat, and an increased consumption of fruits, vegetables and high-fibre cereals. The report stressed the cancer-preventing power of vegetables 'high in carotene which converts to Vitamin A,' thus vindicating Dr Gerson's therapeutic use of large amounts of carrot juice. Also, some American doctors have recently found that old-fashioned porridge, another Gerson favourite, helps to regulate blood sugar and fats, and by lowering blood cholesterol effectively reduces high blood pressure.

We also have the recommendations of the National Research Council of the US on how to reduce cancer incidence. These urge us to cut down our intake of cooking fats and oils, fatty meat, whole milk dairy products, salty, smoked and pickled goods and alcohol. In Britain, the Royal Berkshire Hospital's special diet might have come straight from Dr Gerson's book. It bans salt, salty, smoked and tinned foods, cream, cheese, cakes, fatty meat, fried foods, and so on. That diet is for cardiac patients, but its recommendations are valid for the prevention of a whole range of diseases.

In other words, the time and the scientific climate are right for us to switch to a healthier diet.

Here are the rules in a nutshell:

Cut down on animal fats, oils, margarine, red meat, eggs, dairy produce, salt, sugar, refined carbohydrates (ie white flour, white sugar, and all foods containing them), soft drinks, tea, coffee, alcohol and all types of processed and preserved foods.

Increase your intake of fresh fruit and vegetables, fibre-rich cereals, especially oats. In general, your diet should include a high proportion of natural foods with nothing added and nothing removed (which, by definition, means foods that would go off if kept for any length of time).

Avoid chemicals wherever possible. Use filtered or bottled water for cooking and drinking. Review your use of chemicals in your home – are they really necessary? A fly swat, for instance, is less harmful to your health than a toxic spray. Do not use aluminium or non-stick cookware: enamelled, cast iron or stainless steel pots and pans are best. Avoid fried foods.

Switch over as far as possible to organically grown, ie chemical-free products grown on healthy soil. This is a key rule of Dr Gerson which has not yet been 're-discovered' outside the organic movement. Even so, the number of people who no longer wish to eat poison-saturated produce is growing. Obtaining organic food may take some effort, but supplies are getting easier in many parts of the country. If you have a garden, start growing your own organic stuff. If you have not, or if your soil is too toxic for growing edibles, as it is in many big cities, sprout seeds, pulses and grains on your

316

window-sill; it is a cheap and easy way to secure a daily supply of fresh, pure, organic nutrition.

Include plenty of raw foods in your daily intake. Suitably prepared, most vegetables can be eaten raw. Uncooked foods, at their peak, have a quality of vitality which is lost in cooking. Start meals with a raw salad; end them with fresh fruit instead of sugar-rich and lifeless desserts.

Invest in an inexpensive juicer and get into the habit of drinking a fresh, raw fruit and vegetable juice every day – it is the best natural conditioner and rejuvenator.

This kind of diet is no more expensive than the ordinary kind. In fact, it is likely to be cheaper. Although you will spend more at the greengrocer's, you are bound to make considerable savings on junk foods, sweets, meat, chemical-filled soft drinks, salty snacks, alcohol, and so on.

If your usual diet is very different from the recommended one, give yourself time to make the transition. Habits only have as much strength as we give them ourselves – we tend to cling to our bad habits, not the other way round. And it takes some time for our taste buds to recover from the deadening effect of harshly salty, spicy and synthetic flavours. Motivation matters enormously. If you really wish to improve your health and your resistance to disease, the change-over should not be too bad.

Further Reading

GERSON, MAX, Dr, *A Cancer Therapy – Results of Fifty Cases*, Totality Books, Del Mar, 1977

HAUGHT, S J, *Cancer? Think Curable! The Gerson Therapy*, Gerson Institute, Bonita, 1983

Books on the pyschological approach to cancer:

SIMONTON, CARL, MD, *Getting Well Again*, Bantam Books, New York, 1980

PEARCE, IAN, MD, *The Gate of Healing*, Neville Spearman, Suffolk, 1983

LeSHAN, LAWRENCE, *You Can Fight For Your Life – Emotional Factors in the Treatment of Cancer*, Thorsons, Wellingborough.

Books on nutrition:

GRIGGS, BARBARA, *The Food Factor – Why We Are What We Eat*, Penguin, 1988

KENTON, LESLIE & SUSANNAH, *Raw Energy – Eat Your Way to Radiant Health*, Century/Arrow, 1988

WALKER, C & CANNON, G, *The Food Scandal*, Century/Arrow, 1986

ERLICHMAN, JAMES, *Gluttons for Punishment*, Penguin, 1986

MILLSTONE, E & ABRAHAM, J, *Additives – A Guide for Everyone*, Penguin, 1988

BIRCHER-BENNER, MAX, Dr, *The Prevention of Incurable Disease*, Keats Publishing, 1978

GEAR, ALAN, *The New Organic Food Guide*, Henry Doubleday Research Association, 1988

These books are obtainable from Wholefood, 24 Paddington Street, London W1M 4DR, 01–935 3924

MORE NON-FICTION AVAILABLE FROM
HODDER AND STOUGHTON PAPERBACKS

	BERNARD FALK & ROGER BLACKWOOD	
☐ 48776 8	Why Kill Yourself	£2.99
	TERESA McCLEAN	
☐ 41108 2	Metal Jam	£2.95
	MICHELE ELLIOTT	
☐ 43117 7	Keeping Safe	£2.99
	ANDREW TYLER	
☐ 42273 9	Street Drugs	£4.99
	ELIZABETH WARD	
☐ 42595 9	Timbo: A Struggle for Survival	£2.95
	KATHERINE ADAIR	
☐ 42845 7	Adam: The story of a child with leukaemia	£2.99

All these books are available at your local bookshop or newsagent, or can be ordered direct from the publisher. Just tick the titles you want and fill in the form below.

Prices and availability subject to change without notice.

HODDER AND STOUGHTON PAPERBACKS, P.O. Box 11, Falmouth, Cornwall.

Please send cheque or postal order, and allow the following for postage and packing:

U.K. – 55p for one book, plus 22p for the second book, and 14p for each additional book ordered up to a £1.75 maximum.

B.F.P.O. and EIRE – 55p for the first book, plus 22p for the second book, and 14p per copy for the next 7 books, 8p per book thereafter.

OTHER OVERSEAS CUSTOMERS – £1.00 for the first book, plus 25p per copy for each additional book.

NAME ....

ADDRESS ....

....